Notes on fractures

Notes on fractures

To my daughter Fiona

Notes on fractures

David F. Paton
MB FRCS FRCSE
Consultant Orthopaedic Surgeon,
Whittington Hospital and Royal
Northern Hospital.
Hon. Consultant Orthopaedic Surgeon
The Italian Hospital.
Honorary Senior Clinical Lecturer
Department of Surgery, University College, London.

Churchill Livingstone

EDINBURGH LONDON MELBOURNE AND NEW YORK 1984

CHURCHILL LIVINGSTONE
Medical Division of Longman Group Limited

Distributed in the United States of America by
Churchill Livingstone Inc., 1560 Broadway, New
York, N.Y. 10036, and by associated companies,
branches and representatives throughout the
world.

First published 1984

ISBN 0 443 02864 8

British Library Cataloguing in Publication Data
Paton, David F.
    Notes on fractures. — (Churchill Livingstone medical text)
    1. Fractures
    I. Title
    617'.15   RD101

Library of Congress Cataloging in Publication Data
Paton, David F.
    Notes on fractures.
    (Churchill Livingstone medical text)
    1. Fractures—Treatment—Addresses, essays, lectures.
I. Title. II. Series. [DNLM: 1. Fractures. WE 175 P312n]
RD101.P37 1983 617'.15 83-5300

Printed in Singapore by The Print House (Pte) Ltd

Preface

This book is to teach undergraduate students all they need to know about fractures.

Recognizing that they have a vast amount of factual knowledge to digest, the author has developed a system of teaching which demands the least possible learning by rote.

The undergraduate **must** learn the 'General principles of fracture treatment' (Part I). After this he or she will only be asked to memorize that information which is peculiar or particular to the individual fracture under discussion. It will be taken for granted that the student will apply the general principles already mentioned.

The author makes no apology for directing this booklet towards the requirements of examiners as well as the more important area of adequate management of fractures. The book is based on a system of teaching fractures which the author has used in teaching undergraduates over many years.

London, 1984   D.F.P

Acknowledgements

I wish to thank Mr Martin Lowy for reading through the text and offering many helpful suggestions, the surgeons who taught me and finally the students whose interest stimulated me to write this book.

Contents

Part 1
General principles of fracture treatment

Part 1

Classification

A fracture indicates a complete or partial break in the continuity of a bone. Fractures may be classified in three ways:

I. ACCORDING TO THE CAUSATION OF THE FRACTURE

A. Traumatic fractures
The vast majority of fractures are caused by trauma. The injury may be caused by direct violence, indirect violence or by the violence of muscular pull. Examples of these are:

Direct violence e.g. the ulna is fractured when the arm is put up to ward off a blow with a stick.

Indirect violence e.g. a fall on the outstretched hand may fracture the head of the radius or the clavicle. Here the force is transmitted up the arm.

Muscular pull e.g. the patella may be fractured by a sudden violent contraction of the quadriceps muscle.

B. Stress or fatigue fractures
In these fractures the bone is fatigued by repetitive stress in much the same way as metal fatigues in aircraft e.g. stress fracture of the fibula in athletes.

C. Pathological fractures
A pathological fracture is one in which the fracture occurs through a bone already weakened by underlying disease. Not surprisingly the trauma may be quite trivial or the fracture occur spontaneously. Indeed, this fact may lead the clinician to suspect that the fracture is pathological.

Causes of pathological fractures: General
                                     Local

Generalized disease of skeleton
  1. Disseminated tumours and myelomatosis

2. Osteoporosis — prolonged immobility
   — old age
   — hormonal factors
3. Metabolic conditions — involving metabolism of calcium, phosphorus and vitamin D. Rickets and osteomalacia may result from dietary deficiencies, malabsorbtion from the intestine or loss of salts from renal tubular disease.
4. Adrenal hypercorticalism or excessive steroid therapy.

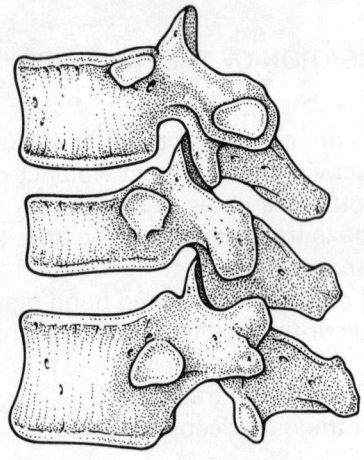

Vertebral body crush fracture typical of metastatic bone disease or osteoporosis

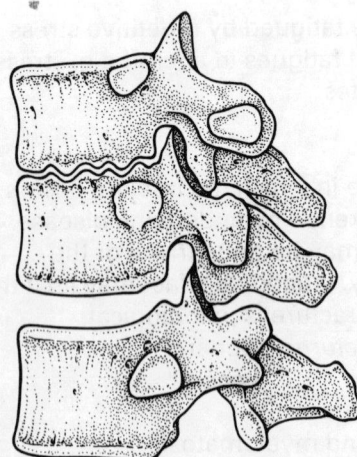

Compare this with the destruction of disc space and adjacent bone which is typical of infection

Fig. 1

5. Hyperparathyroidism.
6. Paget's disease.
7. Neuropathic conditions — syphilis
                                                 — syringomyelia
8. Osteogenesis imperfecta.

Local disease of bone
  1. Metastases in bone from malignant tumours elsewhere. Typically these arise from carcinomata of *breast, prostate, thyroid, kidney* and *bronchus*.
  2. Malignant primary bone tumours.
  3. Benign primary bone tumours.
  4. Hyperaemia and infective decalcification, e.g. osteitis.
  5. Miscellaneous local conditions:
     — simple bone cyst
     — fibrous dysplasia
     — eosinophilic granuloma
     — bone atrophy e.g. polio or meningomyelocoele
     — X-radiation of bone
     — hyatid disease

II. ACCORDING TO THEIR RELATION TO SURROUNDING TISSUES

A. **Simple fractures**
The overlying skin is healthy and closed.

B. **Compound fractures**
The skin has been breached and the fracture site itself exposed to contamination. Note that fractures may also become compound by communication with unsterile body cavities, e.g. air sinuses, mouth etc.

C. **Complicated fractures**
In association with the fracture other important structures have been damaged e.g. nerves, vessels, viscera or joints.

III. ACCORDING TO THE PATTERN OF THE FRACTURE

A. **Complete fractures**
The bone is completely divided into two separate fragments. The fracture line itself may be transverse, oblique or spiral

Often this pattern gives evidence of the nature of the violence and also of the stability of the fracture.

B. Incomplete fractures

1. In children — the bones have an elasticity which permits them to crack and buckle within the periosteal sheath. These are Greenstick fractures.
2. In adults — incomplete fractures are found as the result of impaction. Here the bone fragments have been jammed into each other and are thus stable.

C. Comminuted fractures

There are more than two fragments.

D. Compression or crush fractures

These usually occur in cancellous bone.

Displacement of fragments

The following forces tend to displace a complete fracture: Original violence, muscle pull and gravity. Displacement is described by the movement of the distal fragment on the proximal. Four such displacements are important:

1. *Of alignment*: This refers to a disturbance of the normal longitudinal axis of the bone so as to alter the line through which stress is carried. Restoration of this axis to

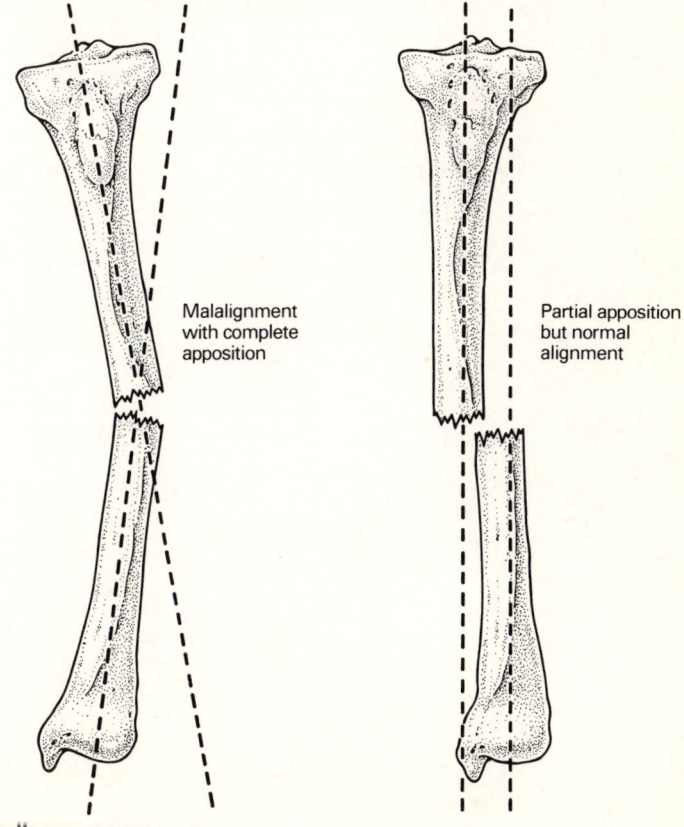

Malalignment with complete apposition

Partial apposition but normal alignment

Fig. 2

normal is important for the continued health of adjacent joints.

2. *Of length:* Shortening can be produced by overlapping of fragments and lengthening by distraction of fragments.

3. *Of apposition*: This refers to the relationship between the bone ends. Ideally this should be complete but union will usually occur even if apposition is incomplete. Note that partial apposition may still permit normal alignment provided that the longitudinal axis of each fragment is parallel to that of the other.

4. *Of rotation:* The distal fragment may rotate on the proximal, about the longitudinal axis of the bone. This displacement should be looked for clinically as it is not easy to see on radiographs.

The diagnosis of a fracture

I. HISTORY

There is a history of trauma. Enquire about the nature of the injury as this information may suggest the type of fracture. If trauma is trivial or absent, consider the possibility of a pathological fracture.

Always enquire about any other injuries. Never forget the possibility of *associated injuries*.

Take a brief general history with attention to establishing the fitness of the patient for anaesthesia. The following points will avoid embarrassing the anaesthetist:

? State of cardiovascular and respiratory systems.
? Presence of diabetes.
? Patient on steroid therapy.
? Patient taking any other drugs or allergic to any drugs.
? Time of last food or drink.

II. EXAMINATION

A. Pain and tenderness are usually present, both over the fracture and on moving the part.
B. Swelling and bruising.
C. Deformity.
D. Abnormal mobility, i.e. movements where no joint exists.
E. Absence of transmitted movements.
F. Loss of function.
G. Crepitus. This may be found incidentally, but should not be deliberately elicited.
H. Discrepancies in length of limbs.
I. A *routine examination to exclude associated injuries*.
J. A *routine examination to exclude complications of fracture*.

A search should be made for wounds indicating that the fracture is compound. The nerves supplying the part concerned should be tested. The blood supply of the limb must be examined. Observe the peripheral pulses, colour of skin, temperature of skin, capillary return etc.

NOTE: When making notes about the examination, it is wise for medicolegal reasons to write down that other injuries and complications have been excluded.

III. RADIOGRAPHIC EXAMINATION

An X-ray should be taken whenever there is the possibility of a fracture. Two films at right angles to each other are usually taken and you should ask for these.

In certain circumstances extra films are of value. Oblique views and comparison films of the normal limb may then be requested, e.g. in suspected fractures of the elbow in children the epiphyses may give rise to diagnostic difficulties. A comparison film of the normal side is of great help.

Radiographs are also used to confirm that reduction has been achieved and subsequently to follow the progress of union.

The healing of fractures

The healing of fractures is in five main stages:

1. **Haematoma formation**

2. **Organization of haematoma**
Within hours of this injury fibroblasts from adjacent tissues begin to enter the haematoma and within a few days capillary buds grow into it. The result is the gradual organization of the haematoma to granulation tissue.

3. **Callus formation**
The fibroblasts in the granulation tissue show metaplasia and change into collagenoblasts, chondroblasts and later to osteoblasts. Osteoblasts from adjacent healthy bone also participate. Bone is laid down in a haphazard fashion around collagen fibres and islets of cartilage. This is called WOVEN BONE. The callus causes the fracture to become firm and may be felt as a mass. It is visible on a radiograph.

4. **Consolidation by mature bone**
The woven bone is replaced by lamellar bone.

5. **Remodelling**
Excess callus is removed and the bone resumes a normal or near normal shape. The medullary canal is recanalized. Children have great powers of remodelling and may correct deformities and even discrepancies of length after a fracture.

TIME NECESSARY FOR UNION

This varies quite widely and differs between one bone and another. However, the following rule of thumb is helpful:
— Cortical bone requires 3 months to heal in adults.
— Cancellous bone requires 6 weeks to heal in adults.
— Children require about half as long as adults.

Principles of fracture treatment

FIRST AID

In principle this consists of measures to limit pain and to prevent further damage by excessive movement of the fragments. Elaborate splintage may cause pain and waste time if the patient does not have far to travel to hospital. Such measures as a sling for upper limb fractures and bandaging to the normal leg in lower limb fractures are simple and effective. Prevent bystanders from giving the patient, 'a nice cup of tea' as he may require an anaesthetic.

Compound fractures should be covered with the cleanest material available. Otherwise treatment is as above.

TREATMENT OF SHOCK

It is important to know that the fracture of a large bone may be associated with considerable blood loss, e.g. 1litre — 1.5 litre of blood may frequently be lost around a fractured femur. Hence in cases with multiple fractures oligaemic shock may be present. Neurogenic shock due to pain may be superadded. Such cases require urgent transfusion with blood or plasma volume expanders.

Beware of sending a patient off to the X-ray department without an intravenous infusion as he may become shocked while not under observation. It is important to add, that adequate doses of analgesics should be given early provided that there are no contraindications.

PRELIMINARY ASSESSMENT

Careful examination is necessary to establish a baseline for subsequent observations. The facts of this examination must then be recorded. It must be emphasised again that *associated injuries* and *complications* of the fracture must be sought and excluded.

AIMS OF TREATMENT OF FRACTURE ITSELF (Fig. 3)

1. *Reduction.* This means the restoration of the displaced fragments to their anatomical position.
2. *Immobilization or fixation.* This means retention of the fragments in the reduced position until union.
3. *Achievement of union.*
4. *Restoration of function.*

Reduction
The decision as to whether a fracture requires reduction or not is one of the main arts of fracture treatment. In general, it may be said that in cases where the displacement is very slight, or where function of the limb may be restored to normal without anatomical reduction, or in children who have greater powers of remodelling, small displacements may be accepted. In general, imperfect alignment is less acceptable than imperfect apposition. It must be repeated that considerable experience is required in these decisions. A fracture that requires manipulation requires an anaesthetic. Local and regional anaesthetics have their place, but a general anaesthetic is desirable in any major fracture as it produces muscle relaxation.

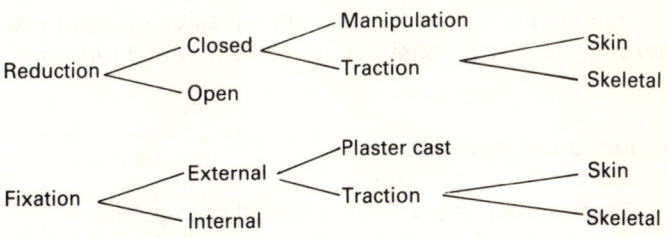

Fig. 3 Summary of methods of fracture treatment

Methods of reduction
1. Manipulative reduction of the fracture with external fixation in a plaster cast.
2. Manipulative reduction and fixation by skin or skeletal traction.
3. Reduction by mechanical traction.
4. Mechanical reduction of the fracture, controlling the fragments and fixing them by skeletal transfixation.

5. Open reduction of the fracture usually with internal fixation, but sometimes with external splintage.

Plaster technique

Students should ensure that they have practised the art of plaster bandaging.

It is advisable always to plaster over a layer of plaster wool.

If considerable swelling is present it may be preferable to use a plaster slab only at first and complete this to a full plaster at a later date.

The position of the fragments should be checked by X–ray in the plaster.

Instructions should be given to outpatients to report any tightness or signs of vascular impairment in the limb.

Every plaster should be checked on the following day.

Indications for traction

1. Where powerful muscles tend to cause shortening or angulation of the fracture, e.g. fracture of femur.
2. Extremely unstable fractures, e.g. oblique fractures which tend to shorten.

Methods of applying traction

Traction may be applied to the skin via adhesive plaster or to the bony fragments by transfixing them with metal pins or wires.

Open reduction of fractures

Indications:

1. Inability to obtain reduction by closed manipulation. This may be due to muscle pull or interposition of soft tissues. Intra-articular fractures may require this to restore articular surfaces.
2. Inability to maintain reduction due to instability of fractures. The fracture may slip after a perfect initial reduction.
3. Some surgeons believe that rigid internal fixation by special plates etc. ensure the best chance of early union. However, if fixation is inadequate, union may, in fact, be delayed by open reduction.
4. Internal fixation permits early mobilization of adjacent

joints, but weight bearing must be delayed until union is well advanced.

The great danger of open reduction is that it converts a simple fracture into a compound fracture and ensuing infection may prove very difficult to eradicate. This risk has often to be taken to ensure a good result.

Optimum time for open reduction
If early reduction is desirable, then the sooner the better is the axiom. However, certain fractures are not disadvantaged if open reduction is delayed for 10 to 14 days, e.g. fracture of the femur.

Methods of internal fixation (Fig. 4)

1. *Suturing with wire or other suture*

2. *Screwing of fracture with stainless steel or alloy screws*

3. *Plating of fracture*
The fracture is splinted internally by use of a plate fastened to both fragments by screws. Recent improvements in design of instrumentation and internal fixation devices have allowed 'rigid' internal fixation. Compression of the bone ends can be added further to improve fixation. Fractures treated by these methods heal well without forming much external callus. There is some doubt whether 'rigid' fixation is always advantageous and very recently 'semi-rigid' plates have been introduced to encourage external callus formation. Occasionally 'double' plating with plates at right angles to each other may be needed for difficult fractures.

4. *Intramedullary nailing*
The passage of an intramedullary nail along a fractured tubular bone can achieve fixation which is mechanically very strong. By careful attention to reaming of the canal quite large nails may be introduced to produce the best possible fixation.

5. *External fixation devices*
Here the fragments are transfixed by pins which are assembled and held in an external fixation device to give very effective immobilisation of the fragments. By careful adjustment of the pins before they are clamped into the

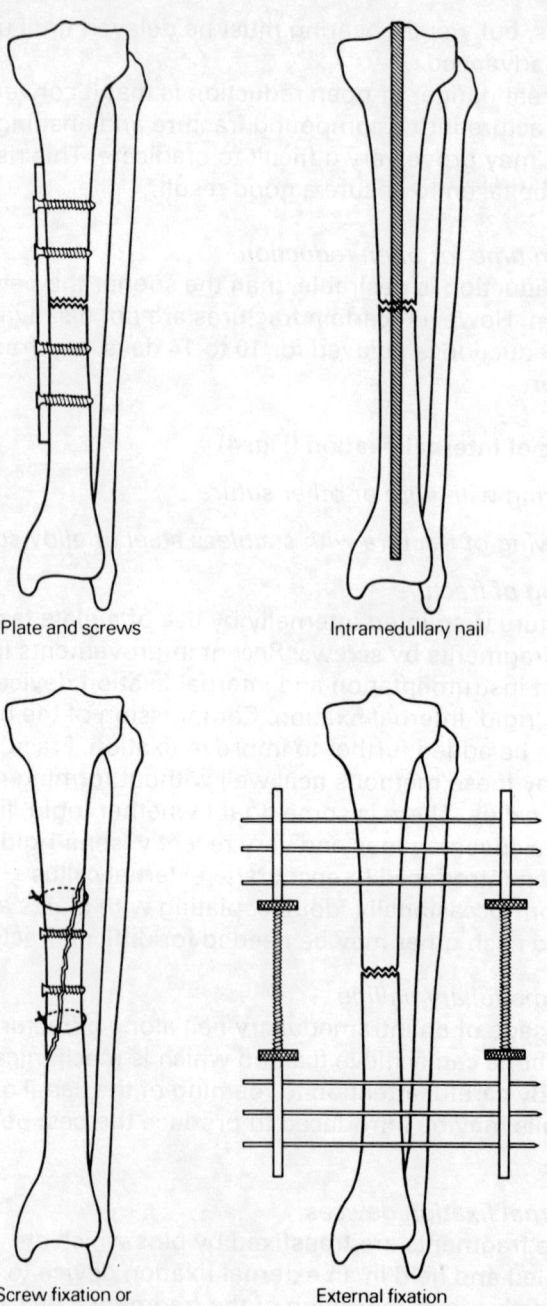

Plate and screws

Intramedullary nail

Screw fixation or
encirclage wiring

External fixation

Fig. 4

fixator, very awkward and comminuted fractures can be reduced and held.

This technique is of special advantage when there is much damage to skin and soft tissues. The fracture can be held while the surgeon has access to the damaged tissues for dressings, skin grafting etc.

Recent improvements in the design and versatility of fixators and the shape of the pins have permitted very efficient fixation of difficult fractures without the loosening and pin track infection which used to bedevil this method.

Restoration of function
The restoration of function of the injured part and the rehabilitation of the patient as a whole is of the greatest importance in the management of fractures. Less dramatic than early surgical procedures, it tends to be forgotten.

Preventative measures
Oedema and subsequent stiffness are closely linked, especially in injuries to the wrist and hand. Where considerable oedema is present, admission to hospital for elevation of the part is desirable. In less severe cases a sling suffices. Similarly, in injuries to the leg, elevation of the part reduces swelling.

All outpatients with fractures must be given specific advice to exercise as much of the injured limb as is accessible, e.g. in a case of Colles fracture the patient must be taught to exercise fingers, elbow and shoulder.

It is not necessary to refer every outpatient for physiotherapy. However, those cases with oedema and early stiffness must be looked for and referred for treatment. Inpatients can usually be supervised, both by the clinician and physiotherapist, but nevertheless advice to exercise on their own should be given.

Active use
As much use of the injured part must be encouraged as is compatible with successful treatment of the fracture.

Active exercises and physiotherapy
Even when a limb is splinted, the muscles must be actively exercised. Static contractions are encouraged. As soon as

rigid splinting is no longer essential, gradual movement of the joints must be encouraged.

Active movements are always preferable to passive stretching. In the elbow, passive stretching can lead to myositis ossificans.

When the fracture is soundly united, treatment is intensified until the part is returned to normal, or near normal.

Return to normal living and employment
The return of the patient to normal daily activities including employment must be the aim of the clinician. The patient may need firm encouragement to return to work. Help may be necessary from employers, occupational therapists, social workers and resettlement officers. If there appears to be any inexplicable delay in return to work, tactful enquiries about litigation may reveal the cause. In these cases the advice of the resettlement or rehabilitation units is often a great help.

Treatment of compound fractures
The object of treatment of a compound fracture is to try to prevent the contaminated wound from becoming infected. Infection leads to osteomyelitis, which may be difficult to eradicate. It may be discussed under the following headings:

1. *First Aid*
(vide supra)

2. *Resuscitation*
In compound fractures blood loss may be external as well as internal but otherwise the basic principles of resuscitation as previously discussed apply.

3. *Preliminary assessment*
(vide supra).

4. *Antibacterial therapy*
Antibiotics should be given as soon as the diagnosis is made. Ideally large doses of suitable antibiotics should be given by intramuscular injection e.g. Benzyl penicillin 1 mega unit six hourly plus flucloxacillin 500 mg six hourly should be adequate in most cases. If the wound is grossly

contaminated, gentamycin should be added with the usual attention to renal function and serum levels where these investigations are available. This treatment should be continued until the clinician is certain that the wound is not infected. Antitetanus precautions must be taken. Human antiserum is now available and should be used in patients who are not presently immunized. Otherwise a tetanus toxoid booster dose may be given. Adequate antibiotic therapy plus surgical cleansing should protect adequately against gas gangrene.

5. *Treatment of wound and of fracture*
Compound fractures require early treatment and operation should not be delayed. The object of treatment is to cleanse the wound, remove all contaminating material and to excise the dead and devitalized tissue. The extent of the wound determines the extent of the surgery. A simple puncture wound may need no more than cleansing and suturing. Any wound where there is a possibility of contamination requires exploration and a surgical toilet.

If necessary, the wound is enlarged. A narrow strip of skin at the margin of the wound, together with any bruised or crushed tags, is excised. All crushed tissue is exposed and the fascia overlying it is incised and laid open.

The wound is thoroughly cleansed with saline or detergent solution and foreign material carefully removed. The emphasis should be on cleansing, rather than excision, of tissue. However, any crushed or devitalized muscle should be excised to prevent infection by gas gangrene organisms.

Small pieces of bone unattached to soft tissue may be picked out, but generally bone fragments should be left.

Damage to major blood vessels is dealt with at the time, but nerves are left for later suture. The ends of severed nerves should be tacked lightly together to facilitate identification later and to prevent retraction.

Skin closure by primary suture, or skin grafting should be attempted with the following exceptions. If contamination has been gross, or if the injury is older than 12 hours, it must be regarded as infected and left open. Packing with sterile gauze encourages drainage. Delayed wound closure may be necessary in such cases.

The matter of internal fixation in compound fractures arouses controversy. In the main, it is thought to be inadvisable to fix a compound fracture internally as the hazard of infection is increased. An exception to this is the case where soft tissue damage is so gross that fixation of the fracture is essential for the survival of the soft tissue. In cases needing arterial repair, fixation is advisable.

Internal fixation may, of course, be performed at a later date when the skin is healed and no evidence of infection exists. The use of external fixation devices may permit awkward compound fractures to be fixed even in the presence of severe soft tissue damage.

6. *After care of compound fracture*
The wound is inspected through a window in the plaster if necessary at about 10 to 14 days. If clean and healed the sutures are removed and further treatment is as for simple fracture. If the wound is infected then treatment is as for osteomyelitis, but union must be the aim of treatment.

The complications of fractures

1. The fracture may be complicated by *associated injuries*.
2. The fracture may be complicated by injuries to nerves, vessels, viscera, joints or ligaments.
3. Complications of fracture itself.

NERVE INJURIES

Primary nerve injuries are caused at the time of the fracture by *contusion*, *stretching* or *division* of the nerve. The term 'neuropraxia' is used to describe a minor injury in which a physiological block is caused and recovery may be expected in a few weeks. The term 'axonotomesis' refers to an injury which damages axons sufficiently to cause peripheral degeneration, but leaves the architecture of the axon tubes undamaged. The axon regenerates at the rate of about 1 mm per day and recovery may thus take months. The term 'neurotomesis' refers to destruction of the whole nerve and subsequent fibrosis defeats efforts at regeneration. Normally excision of the damaged section and suture is required before there can be a chance of recovery in a case of neurotomesis.

In closed fractures, it may be assumed that the lesion is recoverable and treatment is conservative. Physiotherapy to maintain movements in the paralysed joints and splintage to prevent overstretching of the paralysed muscles by functioning antagonist muscles or gravity is necessary.

If recovery does not occur in the expected time exploration of the nerve is advisable.

In open fractures it is usually assumed that the nerve has been divided and exploration and suture are usually performed about four weeks after the injury. If the nerve is found to be in continuity it is left and the wound closed.

Nerves may also be involved later in callus causing a 'secondary nerve injury'.

INJURIES TO BLOOD VESSELS

The vessel may be contused, lacerated or severed.
Superadded *thrombosis* or *spasm* exacerbate the ischaemia.
Arterial spasm may be extensive even when the actual
segment traumatised is quite small and the damage
relatively minor.

Further diminution of the blood supply to the extremity
may be caused by *tension* within the fascial sheath due to
oedema and haemorrhage.

Certain fractures are prone to vascular injuries,
particularly supracondylar fractures of humerus and femur.
An important example of this is the condition of Volkmann's
ischaemic contracture of the forearm. Typically this results
from injuries in the region of the elbow joint in children, the
most common being the supracondylar fracture. The
contracture is the late result of fibrosis of the deep muscles
of the forearm which have undergone ischaemic necrosis.
Indications of ischaemia after injury are:

A. Excessive pain.
B. Absent radial pulse.
C. Pallor or duskiness of the fingers.
D. Poor capillary return.
E. Inability to extend passively the fingers.

The condition is not unknown in the deep muscles of the
calf after tibial fractures, but is less often recognized.

Treatment is an urgent matter and depends upon:

1. If the fracture is as yet unreduced, early reduction is
   essential.
2. If the fracture has been reduced, all constricting
   bandages, plasters etc. must be removed and excessive
   flexion of the elbow relaxed.
3. If this does not help, the lesion must be explored.
   Sometimes division of the fascia alone relieves tension
   and spasm. Hanging the arm over the side of the table
   for 10–15 minutes often restores circulation once the
   fascia has been divided. Occasionally the artery itself
   has to be exposed. Spasm may then be relieved by
   stroking the vessel or bathing it in paraverine solution.

Rarely, excision of the damaged segment is required with
or without repair.

Cooling of the affected limb helps to reduce metabolic
demands.

THE COMPARTMENTAL SYNDROME

In certain fascial compartments muscle ischaemia can arise without there being a major arterial injury. Swelling of muscle occurs and the intracompartmental pressure rises. When the pressure exceeds diastolic pressure then ischaemia commences as a result of small vessel occlusion. Note, however that major vessels passing through the compartment may still transmit pulsation distally until the intracompartmental pressure reaches the systolic blood pressure.

Intracompartmental pressure may arise from a variety of causes. Obviously trauma must be the most important but the condition has been described even as a result of muscle swelling after heavy exercise.

This mechanism plays an important role in the forearm ischaemia described above. Other compartments where this occurs lie in the deep flexors of the calf, the anterior tibial compartment and the peroneal compartment.

It is very important that surgeons should be aware of the existence of compartmental syndrome as this information emphasises the importance of early fasciotomy which is the only way in which this particular source of muscle ischaemia can be relieved.

COMPLICATIONS OF THE FRACTURE ITSELF

1. Delayed union
This is a clinical term which refers to a fracture which does not unite within the expected average time. Treatment is expectant, but there comes a time when the clinician has to regard the delayed union as a case of non union and treat accordingly.

2. Non-union
Here the attempts at repair have come to an end. There is a typical radiological appearance. The bone ends are sclerosed. No trabeculae cross the fracture line which indeed becomes more apparent. The marrow cavity becomes closed. In extreme cases the body attempts to create a false joint or 'pseudarthrosis'.

Causes of non-union
a. Infection.
b. Poor blood supply.
c. Excessive movement at fracture site.
d. Loss of apposition of fragments, particularly distraction.
e. Corrosion of metal used to internally fix the fracture.
f. Interposition of soft tissues between the bone ends.
g. Underlying disease of bone in pathological fractures.

Treatment of non-union
The treatment is by bone grafting with or without internal
fixation. Cortical bone or cancellous bone may be used.
Most frequently today cancellous bone is used packed
between and around the fragments. Clinical reasearch is in
progress to evaluate the use of electrical stimulation of
union in cases of delayed or non-union.

3. **Mal-union**
This term means that the fracture has united in a position of
deformity. This usually indicates a failure of treatment.
Interference with alignment may cause the adjacent joints to
be at a mechanical disadvantage with early ensuing
secondary osteoarthritis. Whether treatment is required or
not depends upon the degree of deformity, age of patient,
fitness for surgery and age of the fracture. If the fracture is
not yet united, deformity may be corrected by manipulation
or wedging of the plaster. When it is united the bone has to
be refractured or divided. In general mal-union affects more
seriously weight bearing joints than non weight bearing
joints.

4. **Joint stiffness**
Intra-articular and peri-articular adhesions limit movements
of the joint affected. Physiotherapy may have to be
continued for long periods, e.g. up to a year, to restore
function. Occasionally a gentle manipulation under
anaesthesia is useful, particularly with intra-articular
adhesions.
  Joint stiffness is much more likely in a joint previously
abnormal than in a normal joint. Hence children often regain
full movements almost immediately, whereas the aged with
their osteoarthritic joints cannot tolerate prolonged
immobilization without becoming stiff.

5. **Pathological ossification**

Post-traumatic ossification, often called 'myositis ossificans', results from ossification in a haematoma beneath periosteum and soft tissues stripped from the bone by the injury. The elbow is the joint most affected, but it is also seen in the quadriceps muscles and anterior to the ankle, occasionally.

Resting the elbow for three weeks after a severe injury, and the avoidance of passive stretchings are the best ways to avoid this.

In the established case, passive movements must be stopped and active exercise continued. If the disability is great, surgical excision of the abnormally situated bone may be performed, but only when it is 'mature'.

6. **Avascular necrosis of bone**

Death of part or the whole of one fragment may result from the cutting off of its blood supply by the accident. This ischaemic necrosis may result in non-union or collapse of the fragment with early osteoarthritis or disorganization of the joint. It usually occurs in sites where the fracture divides the major part of the blood supply to one fragment. The necrotic bone is unable to withstand stress and collapses, often before the process of revascularization can take place.

It may be diagnosed radiologically because the avascular fragment appears more dense on the radiograph than the adjacent bone.

The following sites are most common:

— The head of the femur.

— The proximal half of the carpal scaphoid bone.

— The body of the talus.

— The lunate bone.

There is no specific treatment in the acute stage. In the lower limb weight bearing must be avoided in the hope that healing will occur without deformity. Later surgery is often required for the disorganized joint.

Recognition that this complication can occur is of medicolegal importance

7. **Reflex sympathetic dystrophy** (Eponym: Sudek's osteodystrophy)

This is a condition which occasionally follows sprains or fractures, e.g. Colles fracture. The cause is unknown. Some believe that it is merely severe disuse atrophy of bone, but others believe that there may be temporary abnormality of the sympathetic nervous supply of the limb.

The hand or foot becomes painful, swollen and stiff. It has a reddened, smooth glossy and swollen appearance. Radiographs show a typical patchy osteoporosis.

Treatment requires prolonged, sympathetic but firm physiotherapy. On the whole the prognosis is good.

8. **Osteoarthritis**

This condition may result from an irregularity of the joint surface in any fracture entering a joint, or as a result of the mechanical wear and tear occasioned by functioning adjacent to a malaligned fracture. In the latter case the osteoarthritis may not set in for many years.

9. **Fat embolism**

This condition is a rare complication of major long bone fractures. It is probably more common than is realized, as minor cases are not diagnosed.

Globules of fat from the fracture site enter the venous system and pass through the lungs to the systemic circulation. The fat can cause embolic occlusion of tiny vessels, but it is probable that there is an additional toxic effect as yet not understood. Where the fat comes from is still a matter for controversy.

The clinical features vary slightly as the main effect may be on the brain or on the lungs. They may appear within a few hours to a few days after the fracture.

The patient, who was previously well, may become drowsy and irritable. The pulse and temperature rise, sometimes in bizarre fashion. Petechiae appear on the neck, upper chest, shoulders and axillae in about 20% of cases. In the cerebral type drowsiness may lead to coma and death.

In the pulmonary type the patient becomes cyanosed and develops signs of pulmonary congestion. The PO_2 falls and this is the most useful diagnostic sign in all cases.

The urine and sputum may contain fat globules. X–rays of the chest show a 'misty' appearance in the lung fields.

There is no proven successful treatment and most cases are treated symptomatically. Oxygen therapy with ventilation if necessary may be life saving in severe cases.

10. **Iatrogenic**
a. You may get away with bad treatment of a good fracture or good treatment of a bad fracture but you will scarcely ever get away with bad treatment of a bad fracture.
b. Don't miss associated injuries or complications.
c. Don't let your plasters or splints cause oedema or pressure lesions. Remember the patient is always right if he complains of discomfort.
d. Follow all the rules all the time.

General problems in the management of injuries to elderly patients

1. The patient may be frail and be 'knocked about' by the injury and any anaesthesia or surgery. This may result in confusion and disorientation.
2. The patient may have only just been able to manage by 'tottering' about. The injury may be the last straw and make rehabilitation very difficult.
3. Elderly patients removed from a well known home environment often become confused and disorientated when moved to hospital.
4. Elderly patients tend to lie too still after injuries and are prone to the following conditions:
   — pressure sores
   — bronchopneumonia
   — urinary tract infections
   — fluid and electrolyte disturbances
   — deep vein thrombosis and pulmonary embolism
5. These patients are often osteoporotic to start with and prolonged immobilization aggravates this.
6. These patients are often obese and prolonged immobilization makes them too weak to carry this weight around.
7. These patients are often weak to start with and prolonged immobilization aggravates this.
8. These patients often have pre-existing medical diseases and are generally unfit.
9. 'Disposal' is an ugly word but nevertheless disposal of these patients is often a problem. In uncaring societies the lonely aged often have nowhere to go if they are unable to return home and thus become burdens on available social services.

OSTEOPOROSIS AND OSTEOMALACIA

Elderly persons often have thinner and weaker bones and

are thus more prone to skeletal injury. In this sense such fractures may be regarded as pathological.

There are many causes for osteoporosis but the common variety affecting old people is due to the hormonal changes of later life, particularly in postmenopausal women. It is well known that oestrogen and androgen levels or a combination of the two influence osteoblastic activity. Osteoporosis is the result of failure in the production of adequate amounts of organic bone matrix, osteoid.

Histologically, osteoporotic bone shows thinning of the compacta and widening of the Haversian canals. The trabeculae of cancellous tissue are thin and often distorted by fracture. The ratio of bone mass to medullary soft tissue is greatly decreased and there are considerably fewer osteoblasts than in normal bone.

Radiologically, osteoporotic bones show greater translucency than normal. The cortices are thin and trabeculae fine and rather sparse. There may be pathological fractures such as the commonly seen compression fractures of vertebrae.

The osteoporosis of the elderly may be worsened by disuse atrophy particularly if these patients are confined to bed for a few weeks. Poor teeth or general disinterest in preparing food may result in a diet deficient in protein, calorie intake, calcium and vitamin D so that osteomalacia may add to the weakening of the osteoporotic bones.

Osteomalacia is a condition in which there is an inadequate amount of calcium or phosphorus or both for mineralization of osteoid which is formed to replace bone lost by normal catabolic lysis. In adults the disease may be caused by deficiencies of calcium, phosporus or vitamin D in the diet, disturbances in absorption of calcium or vitamin D from the bowel or excessive loss of serum phosphorus from the kidneys. It is essentially a disease of mineralization and there is no interference with organic matrix formation (c.f. osteoporosis in which there is a deficiency of organic matrix formation). As has been explained the two conditions may coexist.

The disease may be associated with bone pain, pathological fractures and even bone deformity. However, the full blown picture is rare in the Western hemisphere. Milder degrees are however, quite common and the condition should be born in mind in elderly patients with fractures particularly if the fractures are repeated or fail to heal.

Radiographs may be difficult to distinguish from those of osteoporotic patients. The bones are more radiolucent than normal, the trabecular pattern may be coarser and focal areas of radiolucency called pseudofractures or Looser zones may be present. Later the cortices become thinner and less opaque and finally bone deformity and pathological fracture may be seen. The serum calcium or the calcium phosphate ratio may be below normal and the serum alkaline phosphatase is raised. In the last resort the condition may be diagnosed by bone biopsy.

TREATMENT OF THE ELDERLY PATIENT WITH A FRACTURE

In general it is desirable to fix fractures in the elderly internally so that they be kept mobile. Before and after surgery, attention should be paid to maintaining the haemaglobin, fluid and electrolyte balance and to prevention of pulmonary and venous complications. Pre-existing medical conditions may require reassessment and energetic treatment.

Devoted nursing care is essential to maintain their well being, their interest in life and to prevent the many complications to which they are prone.

Rehabilitation of the elderly is often a team effort depending on nursing care, patient but firm physiotherapy, home assessment by occupational therapists, arrangement of social services by social workers and finally help and advice from general practitioners and geriatricians.

Regretably, despite all this effort many patients end up permanently institutionalized.

COMMUNICATION WITH PATIENTS

It always pays the clinician to give a little time to discuss with the patient the likely progress of his injury. This will help him or her to accept the time periods involved, the possibility of certain complicating factors which may lead to an alteration in treatment, and finally, to an understanding of what may reasonably be expected to be achieved after treatment of the injury. e.g.:

A patient with a Colles fracture may be warned that the wrist may not be quite the same shape as before despite adequate reduction, and that there may be a prominence on the ulnar side of the wrist in the region of which some pain may be experienced for a month or two after the plaster is removed.

This kind of communication has the patient on your side during treatment and rehabilitation.

If the injury is a bad one tell the patient early but at the same time give encouragement. Remember it is not your fault that he or she sustained the injury but the patient may be looking around for someone to blame. Hence a poor result may be ascribed by him or her to poor treatment. Adequate and timely communication prevents this kind of unnecessary unpleasantness.

Note

The Author expects students to remember constantly that:
1. Multiple injuries are multiple.
2. The most serious complication of any fracture may be an *associated injury* especially if undiagnosed.
3. Always think of possible complications of fractures and of the treatment of fractures. This will keep you out of trouble with examiners, coroners and patients' solicitors.

Part II
The management of
individual fractures

Part II
The management of
individual fractures

Introduction

If the student has studied and understood the preceding pages, he should have acquired most of the information required to diagnose and treat any individual fracture and also to discuss that individual fracture at an examination.

For example any question concerning fracture of the shaft of the tibia could be answered quite adequately from the information in Part I of this book. As an example let us answer the examination question, *'Discuss fractures of the tibial shaft'* from what we already know:

The fracture may be traumatic or pathological, simple or compound, complete or incomplete, comminuted or even a stress fracture.

The four displacements of the fragments can all occur here. History and examination are as described not forgetting to exclude complications and associated injuries. Radiographic examination in two planes. Time necessary for union — about 12 weeks in adults, half as long in children.

Principles of treatment
— First aid.
— Preliminary assessment.
— Treatment of fracture itself.
— Reduction — all the methods are used at times.
— Plaster technique.
— Indications for traction.
— Open reduction of fractures: indications
                                                 methods.
— Restoration of function: preventive measures
                                            active use
                                            physiotherapy
                                            return to normal living
                                            and employment.

Brief discussion on principles of treatment if fracture were compound.

Complications:
— associated injuries
— injuries to nerves or vessels
— delayed union
— non-union
— mal-union
— joint stiffness
— pathological ossification (rare)
— reflex sympathetic dystrophy
— fat embolism

What an excellent comprehensive answer this would be!

However, if the question were, 'Discuss fracture of the scaphoid bone' the student would require to know some information particular to this fracture. For example:

Caused by falls on the outstretched hand. Tenderness in the anatomical snuffbox. Not necessarily visible on initial X-rays. Requires immobilization in special plaster cast. Prone to non-union and avascular necrosis. Majority of fractures unite if treated adequately but many do not unite if untreated. Non-union may be surprisingly free from symptoms.

It is therefore the purpose of this book in dealing with individual fractures to emphasize that information which is particular to that fracture. The student will be expected to be able to apply the general principles of fracture treatment himself or herself. There will also be paragraphs concerning technical considerations, mainly for postgraduate students, but what the undergraduate student needs to know is the answer to the question, 'What information is particular to this fracture and distinguishes it from other fractures?'

Fractures of the spine

Practical anatomy
The vertebral bodies and intervertebral discs form a strong mobile column well designed to resist compression forces while allowing flexion, extension, lateral flexions and rotation. However, this column is less well constructed to cope with shearing forces either transverse or rotational. Behind the vertebral bodies connected to them by the pedicles are the paired apophyseal joints. These joints together with longitudinal ligaments, and ligamenta flava, interspinous, supraspinous, intertransverse ligaments etc., supported by postural muscles, are the major protection against shearing forces and control rotational stability. These posterior structures may conveniently be named, 'The posterior ligament complex'.

The spinal cord runs in the canal and ends at the lower end of the first lumbar vertebra. Below this is the cauda equina. For a short distance, from about T10-L2, there are roots and spinal cord running together. It is to be noted that a cord transection at the frequently encountered T12-L1 level will isolate the sacral cord below the transection and hence isolate the bladder centre.

The thoracic spine may be regarded as 'protected' against severe injury by the ribs. Hence the areas most vulnerable to rotational shearing forces are near the junctions between 'protected' spine and 'unprotected' spine. In practice this means the thoracolumbar junction and lower cervical spine.

Classification of spinal injuries (Fig. 5)
1. *Classification by mechanism of injury.*
The forces involved are compression, flexion with compression, flexion with rotation and hyperextension.
a. Compression. This usually produces a simple crush fracture.

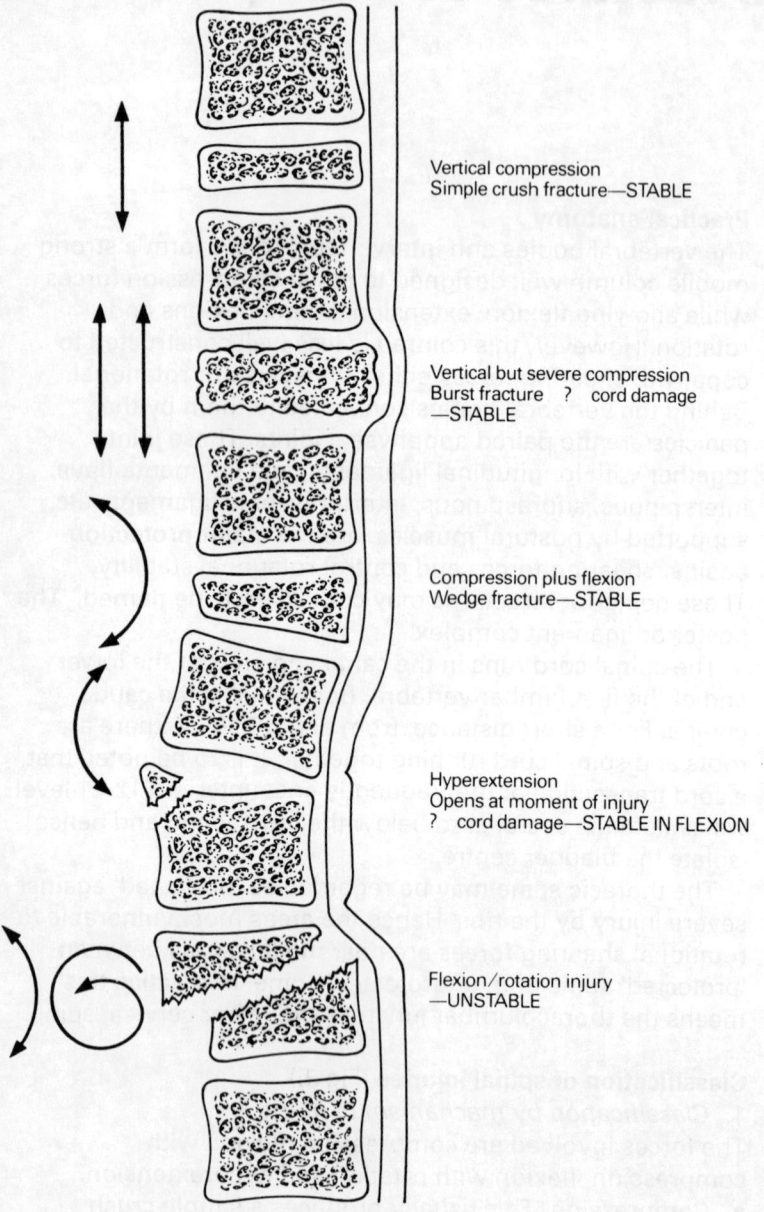

Vertical compression
Simple crush fracture—STABLE

Vertical but severe compression
Burst fracture ? cord damage
—STABLE

Compression plus flexion
Wedge fracture—STABLE

Hyperextension
Opens at moment of injury
? cord damage—STABLE IN FLEXION

Flexion/rotation injury
—UNSTABLE

Fig. 5 Spinal injuries.

b. Flexion/compression. This usually produces a simple wedge fracture.

These fractures are usually stable and innocuous but with excess violence the vertebrae may be virtually 'burst', extruding debris posteriorly into the spinal cord and thus causing cord damage.

c. Flexion/rotation injuries. These produce shearing strains that are likely to produce dislocations and fracture dislocations. In practice this type of injury is the most likely to produce neurological damage.

d. Hyperextension injuries. These are usually caused by a fall onto the face with resulting forced hyperextension of the neck. The displacement is momentary but injury to the spinal cord may be caused.

2. *Classification by stability*
Fractures are either stable or unstable and thus for practical purposes may be regarded as 'safe', 'potentially unsafe' or 'frankly unsafe'.

3. *Classification by association with neurological damage*
Fractures may occur with or without cord or nerve root damage. There is a great difference between the treatment of a fractured spine with cord damage and treatment of a fracture without cord damage.

The significance of neurological damage or instability of the fracture in the management of that fracture
A stable fracture without neurological damage is easily managed. Treatment may be as simple as bed rest or perhaps utilizing a turning bed or even a plaster bed. The point is that the patient can *feel* and therefore does not require constant frequent turning to avoid pressure sores. Such fractures usually heal well with minor after effects such as aching and weakness of the spine.

An unstable fracture without cord damage usually requires more careful attention and some form of immobilization. The cervical spine can be immobilized in a plaster cast, by skull traction with later plaster or by 'halo' splint. The dorsal and lumbar spine can be protected by careful nursing, turning beds or plaster beds. It is rarely necessary to perform opon reduction and internal fixation.

However, persisting instability may necessitate spinal fusion at a later stage.

A fracture with cord damage is treated with the emphasis on the patient with cord damage rather than on the fracture itself.

Spinal shock

After transection, the segmental and intersegmental activity of the cord below the level of the lesion ceases altogether. This is known as spinal shock. After hours or days reflex activity returns in the isolated cord below the transection.

Let us consider by way of illustration a patient admitted to an Accident Department with a fracture dislocation and cord damage in the lower cervical region.

Immediate problems
1. The patient may have an associated injury, e.g. head injuries are often associated.
2. The patient may require resuscitation as result of other injuries.
3. The patient has transected the spinal cord above the sympathetic outflow. There may thus be a precipitous fall in blood pressure.
4. The patient can only survive if he or she can breathe via the diaphragm (phrenic nerve C3-4). This is less efficient and any other respiratory problem recent or past may cause respiratory failure. Even obesity may prove too much of a load.

   The maintenance of an adequate airway when there is an unstable injury of the neck is in itself a problem.
5. The patient may not be able to control body temperature.

Intermediate problems
1. Following successful resuscitation the next problem is that of care of the patient's skin. The patient cannot feel or move and in addition may not be perfusing the skin adequately. This combination may cause pressure necrosis within a few hours. Therefore, two hourly turning of the patient must be commenced as soon as possible preferably within six hours.
2. The bladder. There is no urgency to deal with the paralysed bladder. However, when overflow

incontinence occurs it is time to catheterize the patient. Immaculate technique is necessary to prevent infection which can doom efforts to produce a well functioning automatic bladder.

Our intention must be to drain and keep clean the bladder until automatic reflex activity returns. The ideal outcome if paralysis persists is for the bladder to remain clear of infection and to empty itself regularly when a certain volume of urine is reached. Paraplegic patients are often able to find trick stimuli to precipitate reflex micturition. This is very important to female patients for whom there is no satisfactory incontinence appliance.

Long term problems
1. Careful positioning and bolstering of limbs prevents contractures developing. Physiotherapy maintains joint movement while recovery is awaited.
2. The bowels may become constipated.
3. The permanently paralysed patient has to be rehabilitated as well as possible. In practice independent wheelchair existence is possible if the patient can lift his buttocks off his wheelchair at regular intervals himself or herself. If this is not possible the patient will require 24 hour a day assistance.

   Paraplegic patients often lead very satisfactory and independent lives and can return to useful employment.
4. The paralysed patient suffers from great social, psychological and sexual problems. These have to be dealt with sympathetically.

Care of the fracture itself
Emphasis has already been made towards the significance of sensation in the management of spinal fractures. In most complete cord injuries, sensation will not be present.

Unstable injuries of the cervical spine
These require immediate immobilization. This can be effected by securing a caliper or pair of tongs to the skull. A variety of these exists but the author prefers those which do not require holes to be drilled into the outer table of the skull. The caliper can be applied using local anaesthetic a few centimetres above and behind the ear.

The traction is used firstly to immobilize the fracture. It is applied in the long axis of the body over a pulley attached to the head of the bed. The patient can then be turned in the axis of this traction. If a dislocation of the spine exists with or without a fracture the traction can be used to 'loosen' the dislocation prior to reducing it by manipulation under anaesthesia i.e. unlocking of locked facets. Usually a weight of up to 10 kilograms will be needed to 'unlock' a cervical dislocation. Once reduction has been achieved the weight is reduced.

The traction is maintained for approximately six weeks after which immobilization can be achieved by a variety of methods. The halo splint is very suitable but as the skin over the neck and shoulders usually has sensation, various collars may be used. Patients without cord damage may have the caliper incorporated into a Minerva type of plaster at this stage or be managed safely with this plaster alone.

Spontaneous interbody fusion will often occur within 3–4 months but persisting instability or pain at the fracture site may require cervical spinal fusion which may be carried out anteriorly or posteriorly.

Unstable injuries to the dorsal and lumbar spine
These injuries rarely require internal fixation. The fracture may be satisfactorily treated in the majority of cases by careful turning in a bed or turning frame. Spontaneous interbody fusion usually occurs. If instability or pain persist, spinal fusion may be occasionally required. However, there are certain indications for exploration, reduction and fixation of the fracture internally.

For example, deterioration in the neurological state some time after the injury may necessitate decompression and fixation. A variety of devices may be used to fix these fractures including spinal plates and Harrington rods with laminar wiring.

In general in the U.K. the practice has been conservative. There is a great pressure on the surgeon to 'do something' for the paralysed patient. Unless there is a specific reason for interference, it is wiser to avoid surgery.

Guides to prognosis
There is no certain reliable way of gauging early what the

chances of recovery of a neurological lesion are. Obviously the degree of displacement of the fracture may give a clue. Reflex activity in certain perineal muscles is sometimes a guide. The most encouraging signs are those of incompleteness of the paralysis, or early return of cord function. The patients with early recovery normally achieve the most recovery.

Fractures of the thorax

Although these injuries are often regarded as 'orthopaedic' the important aspects of management are medical.

Rib fractures usually occur as a result of direct violence. They may be very painful and inhibit deep breathing and coughing, thus leading to pulmonary complications, especially in patients already predisposed to these conditions, e.g. elderly chronic bronchitics.

Treatment consists of providing pain relief initially, encouraging breathing exercises as soon as pain allows and observing the patient for complications.

The complications to be thought of and excluded are: Associated injury, e.g. kidney or spleen with lower rib fractures.
— Pneumothorax
— Haemothorax
— Damage to major air passages with surgical emphysema.
— Pneumonia.

Initially the patients will be radiographed. They should be examined clinically from time to time and it is sound practice to repeat the radiograph after a few days to exclude complications.

Pain relief may be difficult. Intercostal nerve blocks may give temporary relief. Strapping the chest in the damaged area only is a time honoured method and affords comfort to some of the patients. Note that the strapping should never extend all around the thorax. This method is probably inadvisable in those patients who are predisposed to pulmonary infection. Most patients will manage with analgesics but pain and tenderness may persist for some weeks.

Multiple fractures of the rib cage, stove-in chest, flail segment

Where there are multiple injuries to the ribs and or sternum the liklihood of contusion and laceration of the lung, penetration of the pleural cavity and injury to air passages increases. Clinically a watch must be kept for air or blood in the pleura and mediastinal shift. Repeated radiographs and blood gas analysis are invaluable in the early phases.

Flail segment injuries of the chest are of particular importance. When a patient inspires, a negative pressure is created in the chest. The first part of the air inspired will come from the dead space. If part of the chest wall is flail i.e. free to move independently, it will be 'sucked in' on inspiration thus occupying space into which the inspired air should have moved. The inward movement of a flail segment when the rest of the chest is moving outward during inspiration is called paradoxical movement.

These patients may of course have additional damage to lung or pleura and may become rapidly anoxic. It is not within the scope of this book to go into the details of management of serious thoracic injuries. However, three actions in the early stages may be life saving.

1. *Endotracheal intubation*. This reduces the dead space, clears the airway and allows suction.
2. *Drainage of the pleural cavities* (with underwater seal). This manoeuvre gives control of the pleural cavities. Now it may be seen if air is escaping into them or whether haemorrhage is occurring. The lungs remain expanded. Also if IPPR is to be used, this may prevent tension pneumothorax.
3. *Intermittent positive pressure respiration*. Ventilation of the patient will cope with most of the eventualities after a chest injury if combined with intubation and pleural drainage. Even flail segments will be controlled.

The management of serious chest injury may be very difficult. Tracheostomy and even rib cage fixation may have a place in individual cases. Antibiotics and physiotherapy play a part. However the three principles above may be life saving as initial measures.

Fractures of the pelvis

Practical anatomy

The pelvis may be likened to a ring, which includes the innominate bones, the sacrum, the sacro-iliac joints and the symphysis pubis. When fractured, the pelvis tends to break the ring at two places (Fig. 6). If only one fracture is visible, consider the possibility of disruption of a sacro-iliac joint (particularly if the patient complains of backache). The pelvis is very vascular and anteriorly the bladder and urethra are positioned vulnerably.

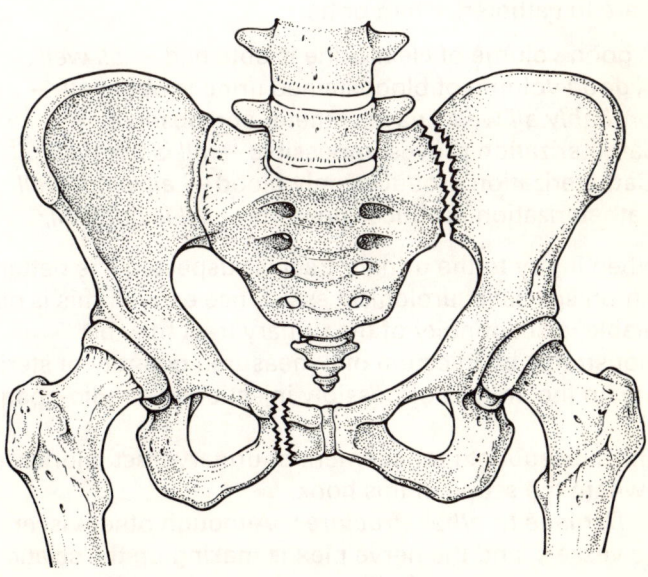

Fig. 6 Typical fracture of pelvis — the 'ring' is broken in two places.

Mechanism of injury

The pelvis is very strong and in most patients a great deal of violence is required to fracture it. Usually this is direct violence of high velocity. As an exception, old ladies with osteoporotic bones may sustain a mild fracture of a single ramus simply by toppling over and crumpling it.

High velocity injuries are often associated with *other injuries* and are often *complicated*.

Early complications and their management

1. *Haemorrhage and shock.* These patients may bleed very severely into soft tissues. Blood loss of 3–4 litres is not uncommon. If the bleeding associated with other injuries is added to this, early severe hypovolaemic shock may be expected. Prepare for urgent replacement of blood loss.

2. *Damage to urinary tract.* Injuries to the urethra and extraperitoneal rupture of the bladder are frequently associated with pelvic fracture. The clinician must establish early that these have not occurred.

The patient is unlikely to be able to pass urine, therefore prepare to catheterize him or her:

a. A good volume of clear urine is obtained — *all well.*
b. A good volume of bloodstained urine is obtained — *probably all well.* Leave catheter and observe.
c. Catheterization proves impossible — *all is not well.*
d. Catheterization produces only blood — *all is not well.*
e. Catheterization produces no urine — *all is not well.*

When injury to the urinary tract is suspected it is better to summon specialist urological assistance early. If this is not available, discontinuity of the urinary tract may be demonstrable by injection of a measured quantity of sterile saline up the urethra or possibly injection of a radio-opaque liquid.

The subsequent management of urinary tract injuries is not within the scope of this book.

3. *Damage to other structures.* Although other viscera, large vessels, and the nerve plexus making up the sciatic nerve are in close proximity, damage to these structures is fortunately rare.

4. *The hip joint.* This is part of the pelvis. Damage to the acetabulum may require treatment.

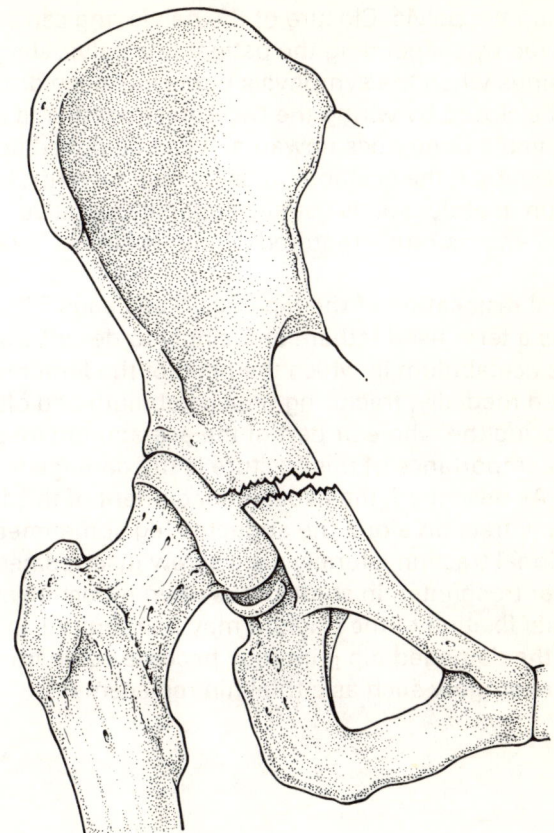

Fig. 7 'Central' dislocation of the hip.

Late complications
These are few. Obstetrical problems rarely arise. A damaged acetabulum may lead to osteoarthritis of the hip.

Management of the fracture itself
You will have noted that this is considerably less important than recognition of and treatment of any complications.

The pelvis tends to open out as a book. Thus placing the patient on a mattress tends to exert a lateral pressure and close up the pelvis. Closure of the pelvic ring can also be achieved by suspending the patient in a pelvic sling. On occasions when the symphysis pubis has been disrupted, it may be closed by wiring the two sides together. If one innominate bone rides upwards, it can be pulled down with leg traction. If the acetabulum is pushed inwards, leg traction in abduction is usually applied. Operative interference is rarely required. Union is almost invariable.

Central dislocation of the hip (Fig. 7: see page 50)
This is a term used rather confusingly to describe a fracture of the acetabulum in which the head of the femur has pushed medially, fracturing the acetabulum and often displacing the whole or part of the acetabulum medially.

The importance of this fracture is the damage to the hip joint. As described, the usual management of this fracture is to apply traction along the abducted leg sometimes with additional traction laterally via a screw inserted near the greater trochanter. In some cases open reduction and internal fixation of the fracture may be required. In the long term the damaged hip joint may become osteoarthritic and require surgery such as a total hip replacement.

The lower limb

DISLOCATION OF THE HIP

Practical anatomy

The hip is a deep socketed joint and considerable violence is required to dislocate it. Not surprisingly associated acetabular fractures are common.

Behind the hip, lies the sciatic nerve in a vulnerable position.

The capsule at the back of the hip which is inevitably ruptured in a dislocation backwards, contains important retinacular vessels supplying the head of the femur.

Mechanism of injury

The majority of dislocations are posterior. They are incurred by an impact on the knee when the patient is in a sitting position, e.g. in a car. The impact on the knee may cause other injuries.

Anterior, inferior and central dislocations also occur but much less commonly.

Diagnosis

The patient has had a severe injury and may have others. Patients with dislocated hips often seem shocked until reduction is achieved.

The affected thigh will be flexed, adducted and internally rotated as might be expected. A history of injury with pain and tenderness completes the picture.

Naturally, the diagnosis is confirmed by a radiograph.
Beware!
We have noted that the injury is caused by an impact on the knee. Hence it is quite common for there to be an associated injury to the patella or femur. A femoral shaft fracture will disguise a dislocation of the hip perhaps leading to one of the great diagnostic disasters of trauma.

It is advisable to insist on a radiograph of the pelvis in all cases with a major injury to the lower limb.

Complications

Early: associated fracture;
        sciatic nerve injury.
Late: avascular necrosis of the femoral head;
        osteoarthrosis of the hip.

Instability in this deep socketed joint is not usually a problem unless there is an associated acetabular or femoral head fracture and therefore recurrence does not occur.

Treatment

The hip must be reduced under general anaesthesia with good muscle relaxation.

It is convenient to anaesthetise the patient on the floor so that the operator may stand over him.

The hip and knee are flexed to a right angle. The deformity is increased and traction is applied in the long axis of the femur. In most cases the hip reduces with a satisfying clunk.

The hip is then rested for six weeks by applying traction to the leg on a Thomas' splint or similar. After this time the patient may be allowed up with crutches non weight bearing on the affected leg for a further six weeks.

If a large bone fragment is displaced from the posterior acetabular margin, open reduction and internal fixation of the fragment may be necessary to ensure stability.

It is advisable to follow these patients as avascular necrosis may appear many months later. Discussion of this possibility may make it easier for the patient to co-operate with the prolonged follow up.

FRACTURES OF THE FEMORAL NECK AND TROCHANTERIC REGION (Fig. 8)

Although there are many differences between these groups of fractures, they share the important common factor of occurring in the same group of patients with the particular problems of that group. They should therefore be considered together.

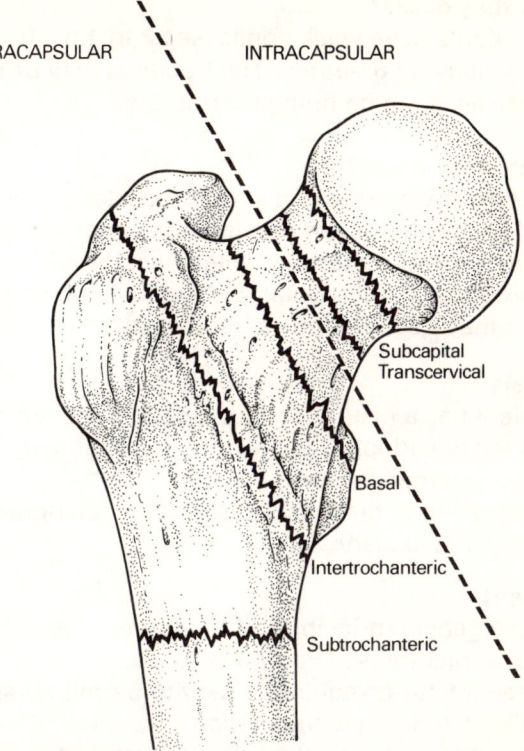

EXTRACAPSULAR   INTRACAPSULAR

Subcapital
Transcervical

Basal

Intertrochanteric

Subtrochanteric

Fig. 8 The sites of fracture of the femoral neck are easy to remember — the descriptions are anatomical. Note that treatment depends on whether the fracture is intra-or extracapsular.

Practical anatomy

The blood supply to the femoral head arrives via three possible routes, in retinacular vessels travelling in the posterior capsule, via medullary vessels in the femoral neck itself and through the ligamentum teres. Of these the first two are much more important and both sources can be damaged when a fracture occurs across the femoral neck.

Note that extracapsular fractures do not damage the blood supply to the femoral head and therefore do not suffer the consequent problems of avascular necrosis of the femoral head and non union.

Who gets them?

These are fractures of the elderly, particularly elderly females.

Why do they occur?
These patients have weak bones (see Part 1 p. 28), and they are less steady on their feet. The fractures may be regarded in a sense as being pathological fractures.

Where do they occur?
The accompanying diagram shows the sites at which femoral neck and trochanteric fractures commonly occur.

Subtrochanteric, intertrochanteric and basal fractures may be regarded as extracapsular. Subcapital and transcervical fractures may be regarded as intracapsular.

Diagnosis
The patient has a history of injury, pain in the region of the hip and the leg adopts a characteristic posture. It appears short and externally rotated.

Confirmation of diagnosis depends on radiographs, preferably in two planes.

Treatment
1. Apply general principles of treatment of elderly patients with a fracture (see Part I p. 30).
2. These fractures require surgery to permit nursing, early mobilization and rehabilitation.
3. In younger patients, (less than 60 years) it is probably advisable to try to conserve the patient's femoral head and pin the fracture.
4. In older patients, pin the fractures which are extracapsular and replace the femoral head of all displaced fractures which are intracapsular. Undisplaced intracapsular fractures may be pinned.

Noteworthy complications
1. Complications of an elderly hospitalised patient undergoing surgery.
2. Avascular necrosis of the femoral head.
3. Non-union of the fracture.
4. Mal-union with varus angulation and shortening.

Technical considerations
A great deal of thought and ingenuity has been devoted to the internal fixation of femoral neck fractures and many methods are available.

Extracapsular fractures require some form of nail and plate fixation. Recently there has been increased enthusiasm for fixed angle nail-plates with compression devices on the nail.

Intracapsular fractures may be pinned in selected cases. Again a nail plate is preferred.

Intracapsular fractures with displacement may require replacement of the femoral head. An Austen-Moore type prosthesis which is punched into the upper end of the femur after reaming may be used. However, a case can be made out for primary total hip replacement in such cases, particularly if the patient is relatively young and fit.

Impacted abduction fractures may be treated conservatively or pinned. It is preferable to pin these with several smaller pins 'spread' into the femoral head. The use of these avoids the danger of displacing the impaction. Serial radiographs should be taken to ensure that disimpaction does not occur. Weight bearing may commence early.

FRACTURE OF THE GREATER TROCHANTER

This injury is of much less importance than the preceding fractures. It may be treated by a period of rest followed by gentle mobilization.

Radiographs may be difficult to interpret and it is probably advisable to repeat the radiographs after a few days in any case where there is doubt as to whether the fracture extends more widely.

FRACTURES OF THE FEMORAL SHAFT

In general terms these are unremarkable fractures and general principles apply:
  1. These fractures occur at any age.
  2 They are usually the result of severe violence.
  3. They may occur at any site and of variable pattern.
  4. Complications are as might be expected after study of Part I. However the complication of fat embolism, fortunately rare, is most often seen after this fracture.
  5. The fracture is most widely treated by manipulation and traction on a splint. *The student must know what a*

Thomas' splint looks like and how it is used. Internal fixation is also often used in management of this fracture.
6. Union usually occurs in 3–4 months.
7. Rehabilitation with exercise is commenced while on the splint and continued more vigorously when splintage is removed.

Technical considerations
   1. *Traction.* (Fig. 9) In children traction may be administered by skin traction and may be balanced or fixed.

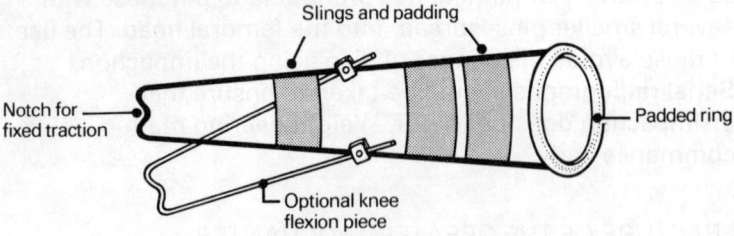

The Thomas splint

Slings and padding

Notch for fixed traction

Padded ring

Optional knee flexion piece

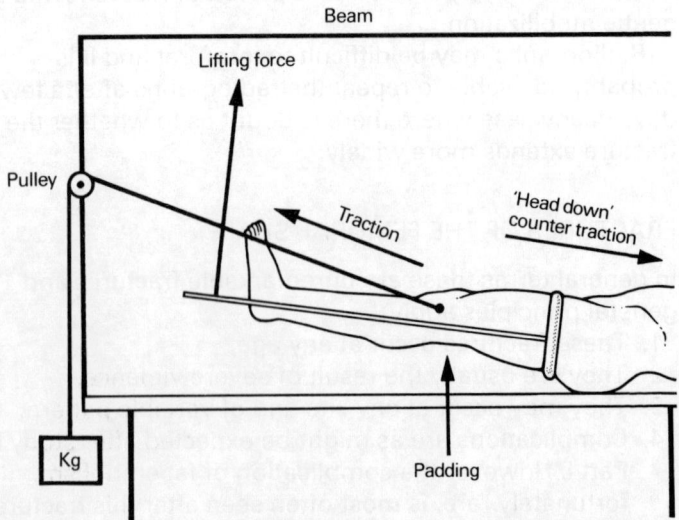

Beam

Lifting force

Pulley

Traction

'Head down' counter traction

Kg

Padding

Fig. 9 The diagram shows sliding (balanced) traction in use but fixed traction — pulling the leg against the ring — can also be used.

Fixed traction is applied from the end of the Thomas' splint against the ring. Balanced traction is usually applied through a skeletal transfixation pin and is taken over the foot of the bed via a pulley as is shown in the accompanying diagram.

In small children under 3 years, Gallows traction may be used from an overhead beam.

2. Once the fracture is 'sticky' external fixation may be used. Traditionally a plaster spica has been the method of choice but more recently widespread use of the method of cast-bracing has been made with considerable benefits to the mobility of the patient. Whichever method is used may permit the complication of late varus angulation and a watch should be kept for this.

3. Internal fixation is possible by a variety of methods. Ideally intramedullary nailing after an accurate reaming of the fragments would be preferred but double plating, single plating and even circumferential banding may be required depending on the shape and size of the fracture.

SUPRACONDYLAR FRACTURE OF THE FEMUR

Practical anatomy
Injuries in region of knee and elbow may damage large vessels.

The gastrocnemii tend to pull backwards the distal fragment (Fig. 10). Therefore immobilization of the fracture with the knee in flexion is desirable.

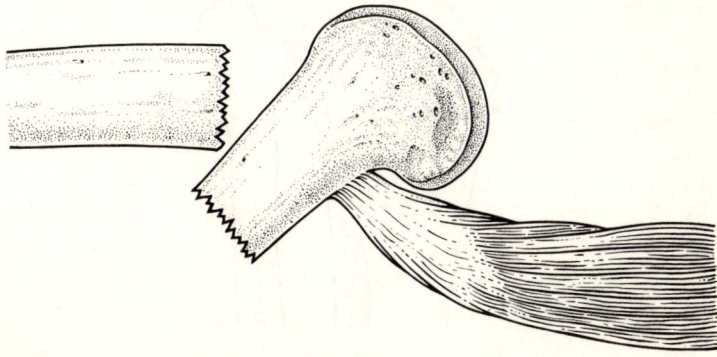

Fig. 10 In supracondylar fractures of the knee, the distal fragment is often tilted backwards by the gastronemii.

Treatment
On the whole these fractures do better with conservative treatment on a Thomas splint with a knee flexion piece added. Internal fixation is possible and may sometimes be indicated.

FRACTURES INVOLVING THE KNEE JOINT (Fig. 11)

Practical anatomy
1. The proximity of the important vessels and nerves behind the knee joint has already been mentioned. *Beware.*

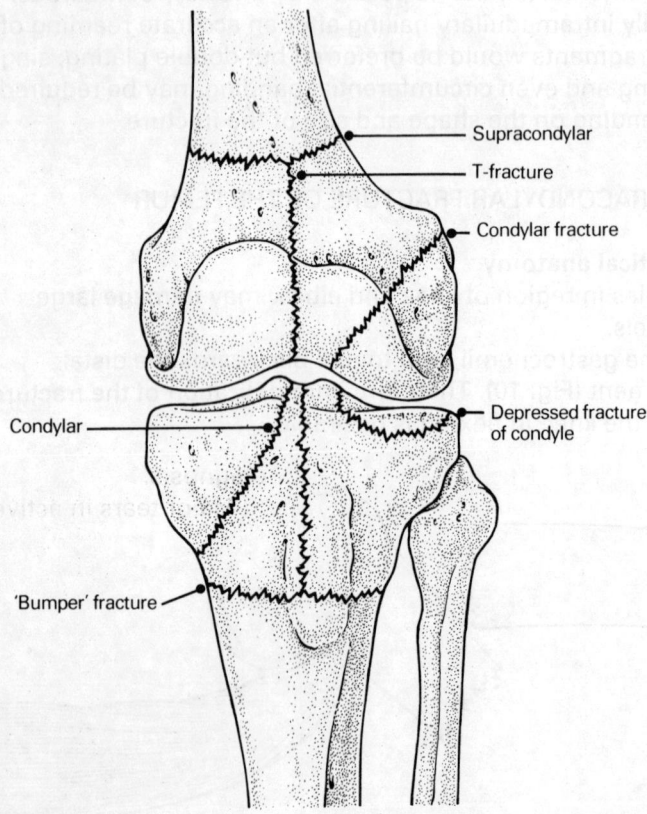

Supracondylar

T-fracture

Condylar fracture

Depressed fracture of condyle

Condylar

'Bumper' fracture

Fig. 11 Fractures around the knee.

2. Weight bearing joints do not tolerate damage or irregularities of articular surfaces well and degenerative disease follows serious injury.

Treatment
1. Painful haemarthrosis may need aspiration for relief of pain.
2. Fractures without displacement or with minor displacement do not require internal fixation. Immobilize appropriately the femur on a Thomas' splint or the tibia in a long leg plaster cast.
3. Minimally displaced fractures of the tibia may alternatively be treated by mobilization while on traction. This ensures early return to full function.
4. Seriously displaced fractures involving articular surfaces need open reduction and internal fixation.

DISLOCATION OF THE KNEE

This is a rare injury. Reduction and immobilization in a plaster cast is adequate. This severe injury is likely to be followed by permanent disability. Beware vascular or peripheral nerve injury. Ligamentous damage is severe. Occasionally immediate surgical repair may be indicated.

FRACTURES OF THE PATELLA

Practical anatomy
1. The patella lies in the centre of the extensor mechanism. It acts as a pulley carrying the mechanism around the knee during flexion. On each side lie the extensor expansions. The patella is thus surrounded by a fibrotendonous 'capsule'.
2. The patella may be fractured by direct violence or by muscle pull or both together.

Treatment
This depends upon whether the extensor mechanism is intact and also upon the degree of comminution of the fracture.

If the extensor mechanism is intact the fractured patella will still retain its 'capsule' and may thus be treated conservatively unless it is severely comminuted. A plaster cylinder is the usual method of splintage.

If the extensor mechanism is ruptured surgical repair with or without patellectomy is essential. In general if the extensor mechanism has to be repaired it is preferabe to retain the patella as patellectomy with extensor mechanism repair is often followed by stiffness.

Severely comminuted fractures with displacement of fragments usually require excision of the patella.

A painful tense haemarthrosis may require aspiration for pain relief.

Other injuries of the extensor mechanism (Fig. 12)
In addition to disruption through the patella and extensor

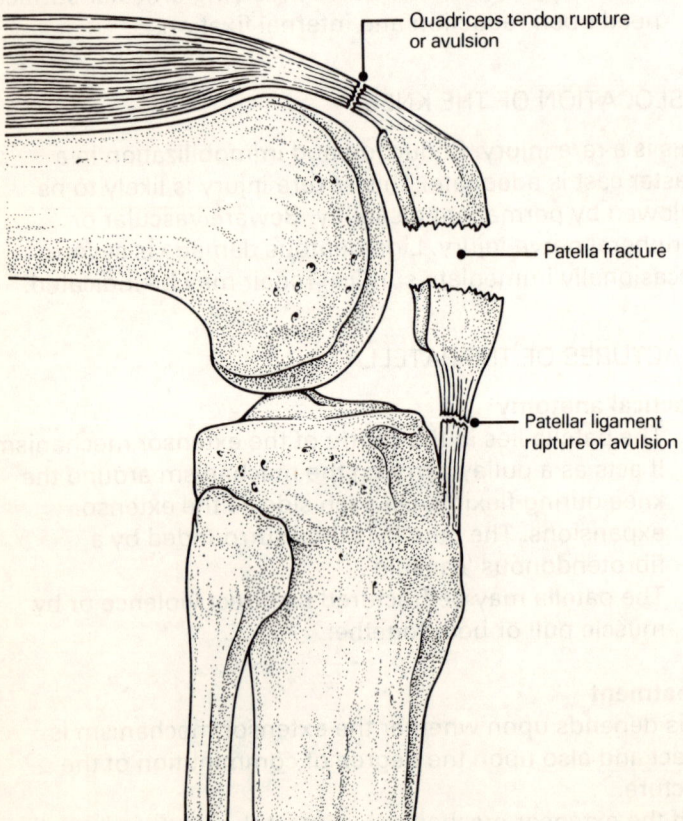

Quadriceps tendon rupture or avulsion

Patella fracture

Patellar ligament rupture or avulsion

Fig. 12 Injuries to the extensor mechanism of the knee.

expansions the extensor mechanism may be disrupted by avulsion of the quadriceps tendon from the patella, by avulsion of the patellar tendon from the tibial tuberosity or occasionally by rupture of the tendons themselves.

Most cases require surgical repair but some elderly patients may rupture the central part of the quadriceps tendon while retaining the expansion intact. In such cases conservative treatment may be justified.

Lateral dislocation of the patella
This condition may occur singly or as a recurrent problem. It is often associated with some other abnormality such as genu valgum, hypermobile or high patella and shallow intercondylar groove on the femur.

The acute condition is quite dramatic as the patella is visibly displaced. It can be reduced by medial pressure while the knee is gently straightened. The torn medial expansion requires resting in a plaster after which vigorous quadriceps exercises are to be encouraged.

Recurrent dislocation requires surgical treatment, the description of which is not within the scope of this book.

FRACTURES OF THE TIBIAL SHAFT

From the students point of view, these are common but unremarkable fractures. General principles apply as was demonstrated on the opening pages (pp 35–36) of Part II.

Technical considerations
Considerable thought, experiment and effort have been expended over the last decade concerning the best way of managing tibial fractures. It must be said that excellent results are being achieved by completely different methods. A simplified guide to the use of available methods is as follows:

1. Transverse, undisplaced or stable fractures can usually be treated *conservatively in a long leg plaster* (Fig. 13). If manipulation is needed, the author prefers to do this while allowing the leg to hang over the end of the operating table. Gravity now assists maintenance of position of the fragments. Dorsiflexion of the foot must be achieved by traction on the heel and not by forcing up the forefoot,

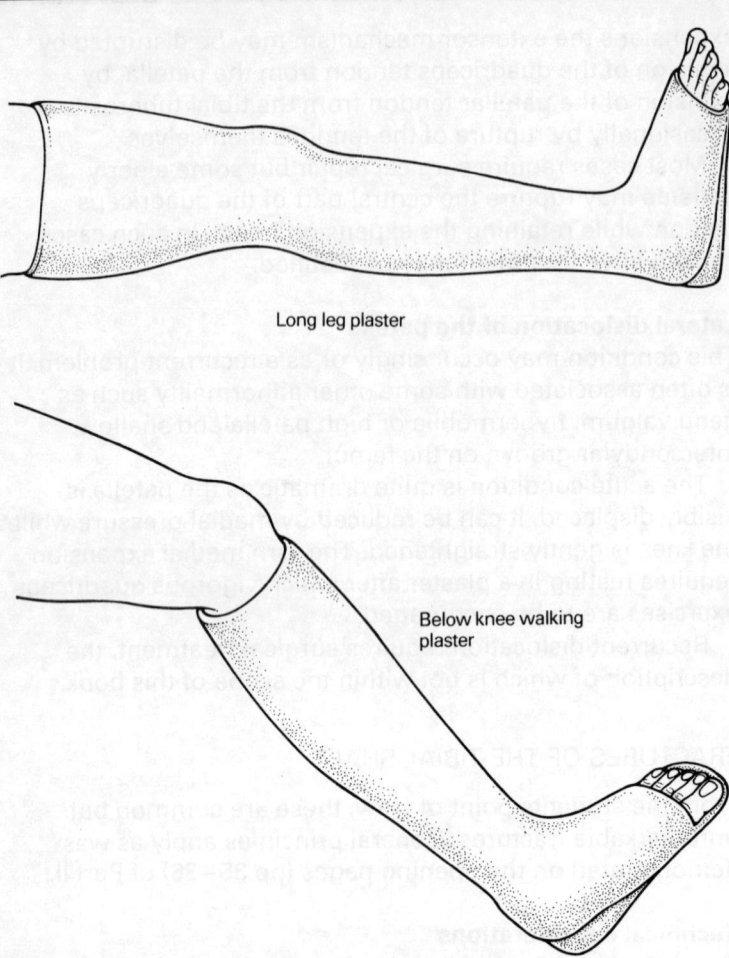

Long leg plaster

Below knee walking
plaster

Fig. 13

otherwise the distal tibial fragment will inevitably tilt
backwards. While the leg is so held an assistant applies a
plaster cast below the knee. The knee is extended and the
plaster cast is completed to an above knee plaster,
preferably with the knee slightly flexed. The ankle should be
at a right angle.

   2. *Traction by calcaneal pin* (or lower tibial pin)
incorporated in the plaster cast may be used for oblique or

unstable fractures. The pin may be cut and buried in the plaster at three weeks and removed with a change of plaster at six weeks.

3. *Rigid internal fixation by plating with or without compression.* This is a successful method provided rigidity is achieved. Not all fractures allow this, in which case the heavy plates and long incisions used are not advantageous.

4. *Semi-rigid fixation with slightly flexible plates of plastic material.* This has recently been introduced to encourage callus formation at the fracture.

5. *Intramedullary nailing* is an excellent method in practised hands for suitable fractures.

6. *Use of external fixators.* This is a useful method when considerable soft tissue damage is present. Whether its use is justified for simple fractures is doubtful. However, transfixation pins of greater diameter and with tapering seem to remove much of the problem of loosening and pin track infection. If these problems can be overcome with more modern devices, then the method of external fixation may be used more widely for fractures unsuitable for conservative treatment.

ISOLATED FRACTURES OF THE FIBULA

This is an uncommon injury as fibular fracture is more commonly associated with tibial fractures or ankle fractures. However, it can occur as a result of direct violence. In general it is an injury not requiring much more than sufficient support to relieve pain. Often strapping will suffice but a below knee plaster can always be used if pain is severe.

Beware of overlooking the combination of a fibular fracture with diastasis of the ankle.

STRESS FRACTURES OF TIBIA AND FIBULA

Both these bones are the sites of stress fractures. These usually occur in athletes who are training over long distances. The gradual onset of pain and tenderness should make the advising surgeon think of this condition and to search appropriate radiographs for evidence of a hairline crack or for endosteal or exosteal callus.

FRACTURES OF THE ANKLE

Practical anatomy

1. The ankle may be regarded as a ring-like structure composed of bones joined together by ligaments. As a general principle instability results when the ring is broken in two places whether as a result of two fractures or a combination of fractures and ligament damage.
2. The commonest way in which ankles are damaged is by inversion injuries. It is everyone's experience to have turned their ankle at some time or other. What is more difficult to understand is that inversion of the foot is obligatorily linked mechanically with external rotation of the talus. When the tibia is held proximally by postural muscles in such a way that it cannot rotate with the talus, then injuries to the ankle mortice may occur. This is the reason that inversion injuries are classified as 'external rotation injuries'.
3. As a general principle a traction force on a malleolus results in a transverse fracture and a pulsion or rotation/pulsion force results in an oblique or spiral fracture of that malleolus.

A simplified classification of fractures of the ankle

1. *External rotation injuries.*   As explained the talus rotates externally driving against the lateral malleolus.

The mildest injury is a 'sprained' ankle with damage to the anterior part of the lateral ligament. Further rotation may fracture the lateral malleolus of the ankle — the commonest ankle fracture apart from minor avulsion flake fractures. If the force progresses, the medial malleolus may be pulled off leading to a bimalleolar fracture or the medial ligament may be torn. We now have an unstable injury.

Continuation of the rotation may cause a fracture dislocation. If the posterior marginal fragment of the articular surface of the tibia is also fractured we have a trimalleolar fracture dislocation of the ankle and this is the true Pott's fracture (Fig. 14).

2. *Adduction fractures* (Fig. 14). Here the foot is fixed and the talus drives medially knocking off the medial malleolus and pulling off the lateral.

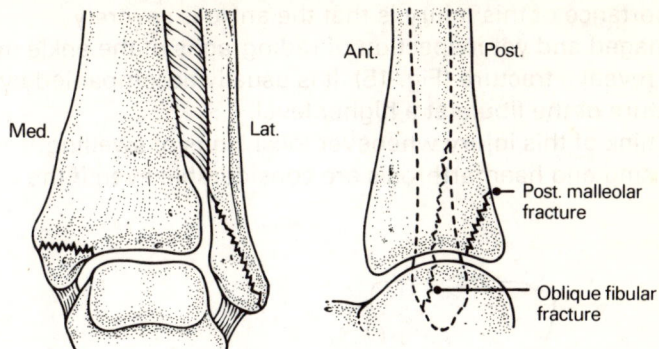

The Potts fracture (External rotation injury)

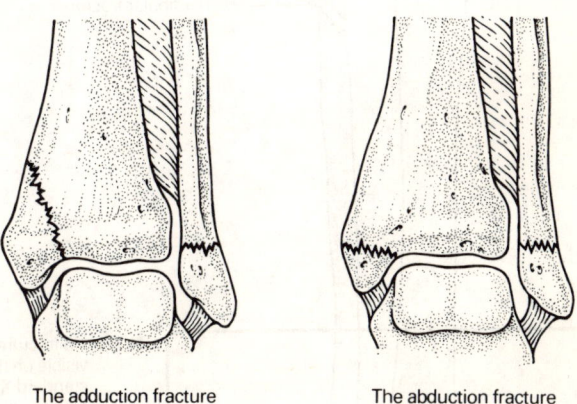

The adduction fracture   The abduction fracture

Fig. 14

3. *Abduction fractures* (Fig. 14). Here the foot is fixed and the talus drives laterally. This fracture bends the rules as both malleoli tend to shear off at joint level.

4. *Vertical compression fracture.* This is really a fracture of the lower end of the tibia involving the articular surface. As a result these fractures are difficult to manage and do badly.

5. *Diastasis of the inferior tibiofibular joint with rupture of the interosseous tibiofibular ligament*. This injury occurs probably as a variation of an external rotation injury. The

importance of this injury is that the ankle is severely damaged and yet inspection of radiographs of the ankle may not reveal a fracture (Fig. 15). It is usually accompanied by a fracture of the fibula at a higher level.

Think of this injury whenever local signs of swelling, bruising and haemarthrosis are considerable even if the

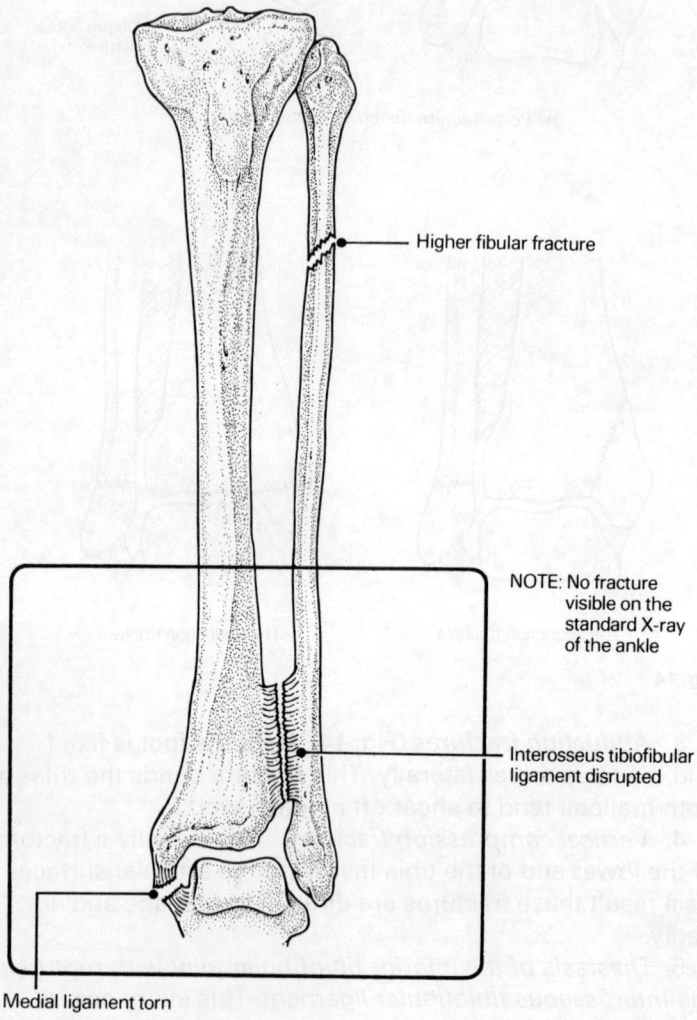

Higher fibular fracture

NOTE: No fracture visible on the standard X-ray of the ankle

Interosseus tibiofibular ligament disrupted

Medial ligament torn

Fig. 15 The diagnostic pitfall fracture.

radiograph shows no fracture. Examine the radiographs closely for signs of widening of the mortice and palpate the whole of the fibula. If in doubt strain X-rays or examination under anaesthesia may be performed.

This is one of the commonest diagnostic errors from accident and emergency departments. Failure to treat energetically an ankle disrupted by diastasis leads to a very poor result.

Look at the diagram and beware!

Treatment of ankle fractures

It is essential to restore as nearly as possible a normal ankle mortice. Failure to do this results in pain, instability and the early onset of osteoarthrosis.

The first essential is to diagnose the injury. The importance of marked swelling and bruising with tenderness on both sides of the ankle has already been mentioned. Radiographs in two planes will show most fractures and usually show evidence of any diastasis. Routine palpation of the fibula takes little extra time.

Stable ankle fractures may be treated conservatively in a below knee walking plaster usually for about six weeks.

Unstable ankle fractures may be treated conservatively or operatively. If treated conservatively then it is the duty of the attending surgeon to follow these cases carefully with serial radiographs to ensure that displacement does not occur as swelling subsides. Use of an above knee plaster cast may be advisable. Weight bearing must be avoided for four to six weeks.

Many surgeons prefer internal fixation for unstable fractures. This should ensure adequate reconstruction of the ankle and prevent late displacement. Although early weight bearing is still not permitted by internal fixation, mobilization of the ankle while avoiding weight bearing may be started after a few days.

Technical considerations

1. *Plaster of Paris* is still widely used for walking plasters. If allowed to dry for 48 hours it is normally adequate. However weight bearing often causes crumpling of the cast. There is a variety of alternative materials available either to replace plaster or to be used to strengthen

it. This is one of the sites where the additional strength justifies the additional expense involved in their use.

2. *Malleoli* may be internally fixed by *screw fixation or* by *tension band wiring.* If screws are utilized it is preferable to use a malleolar screw designed for the purpose. However, almost any screw may be used provided the malleolar fragment is overdrilled i.e. by a larger drill than the screw so that compression may be achieved.

3. In cases where a *diastasis* is present, the mortice should be closed with *a transverse closing screw.* Care must be taken to tighten this with the ankle dorsiflexed so as to avoid overclosing the mortice.

4. *Posterior malleolar fractures may be left alone* if they are small. Certainly any fragment involving a third of the articular surface or more requires open reduction and fixation.

5. *Fibular fractures* may need *internal fixation* to avoid shortening. This may be by plating, screw fixation, intramedullary rodding or by circumferential wiring.

6. If satisfactory internal fixation is achieved the ankle can be mobilized early, but of course weight bearing is not permitted. Once the ankle is moving well a plaster cast may be applied to protect it in the knowledge that mobilization can be more easily achieved later. Otherwise the ankle is usually immobilized until union is well advanced. Early mobilization of the joint in hospital with the limb elevated is ideal but consideration has to be given to bed availability and the facilities available.

FRACTURES OF THE TALUS

These are rare. The important fact to know about these fractures is that the talus receives it blood supply from distal to proximal. Hence a fracture across the neck of the talus may be followed by the expected problems of non-union and avascular necrosis.

Displaced fractures always require open reduction and internal fixation. Undisplaced fractures may be treated in a below knee plaster. Weight bearing should be avoided until union has occurred and no sign of avascular necrosis is to be seen. However mobilization can be commenced earlier.

FRACTURES OF THE OS CALCIS

The calcaneum is like a chicken's egg, strong when intact but crumples under pressure when cracked.

The calcaneum is usually fractured in a fall from a height. Therefore similar compression injuries may occur elsewhere. Look for and exclude in particular crush fractures of the spine.

The subtalar joint is very complex and it is virtually impossible to achieve full movements of this joint after a fracture of the calcaneum. Hence the aim of treatment is to ensure that the ankle does not become stiff.

The ideal treatment is to rest the patient with the foot elevated and to exercise the ankle from the start. When ankle movements are good and swelling settled, the patient may be allowed up, non weight bearing on crutches. This avoidance of load may be necessary for as long as 10 weeks.

Complications include pain and stiffness at the subtalar joint or spreading of the calcaneum which then abuts on the lateral malleolus.

INJURIES OF THE FOOT

General principles apply here. In most cases conservative management is possible utilizing a plaster cast as for ankle injuries. Dislocations must be reduced and held for six to eight weeks. Irreducible dislocations may require open reduction and fixation.

Fractures of smaller toes require treatment only by the wearing of a strong shoe. Crush injuries of the hallux are common. Sometimes a plaster cast is the most useful treatment and occasionally release of a subungual haematoma may afford great relief of pain.

FRACTURE OF THE BASE OF THE FIFTH METATARSAL

This injury is worth special mention due to its frequency.

Here the common inversion injury is combined with forced plantar flexion at the ankle e.g. misstepping on the edge of a step, stair or pavement edge. The peroneus brevis tendon pulls off the 'styloid' base of the metatarsal bone.

Although the injury appears a minor one, there is often soft tissue damage on the dorsum of the foot and a period of immobilization in a plaster cast is often the surest way to achieve a good result.

STRESS FRACTURES OF THE METATARSAL BONES (MARCH FRACTURE)

Metatarsal bones are another site for stress or fatigue fractures. Typically the shaft or neck of the second or third metatarsal bone is affected.

The patient usually gives a history of prolonged exercise. There is a gradual onset of pain in the forefoot. Local tenderness and swelling on the dorsum of the foot are usually found.

Radiographs often do not show the fracture initially but if repeated will demonstrate the appearance of a haze of callus at the fracture site.

If pain is severe the patient may require a below knee walking plaster (Fig. 13) but mild cases require only a period of rest of the part.

The upper limb

FRACTURE OF THE CLAVICLE

Fractures of the clavicle are unremarkable. They may be caused by direct violence but the majority result from indirect violence, a fall on hand or elbow. They may occur anywhere but usually between the middle and outer third. A smaller number occur at the outer end. Complications are few.

They are treated conservatively by bandaging the shoulders into a 'braced back' position. Traditionally a figure-of-eight bandage is used. Care should be taken to protect the axilla with padding. Union usually occurs in adults within three weeks leaving a visible 'bump' at the fracture site (Fig. 16). Warning the patient about the expected 'bump' ensures good relations.

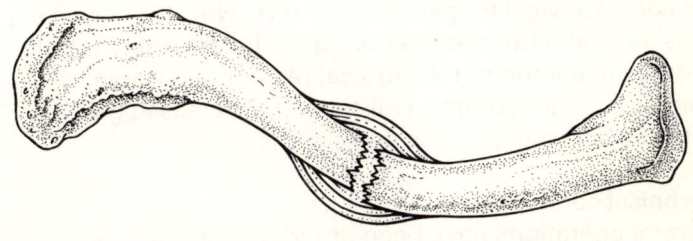

Fig. 16 The fractured clavicle often heals with a 'bump'.

FRACTURES AROUND THE SHOULDER

Practical anatomy
Learn to feel the bony points of your own shoulder. Note
that the head of the humerus forms the rounded curve of the
shoulder. Note also that it is remarkably anterior. The
coracoid process can be felt medial to the humerus and the
acromion process above it. The acromio-clavicular joint can
just be felt. Behind the shoulder can be felt the spine of the
scapula with the infra-spinous and supraspinous fossae.

FRACTURES OF THE SCAPULA

Fractures of the scapula are usually due to direct violence
and soft tissue bruising may be extensive. Fractures of the
body and neck are usually little displaced because of
splintage by attached muscles.

Treatment is by rest, analgesia and mobilization as soon
as pain permits. Occasionally a displaced fractured acromion
process needs to be excised.

INJURIES TO THE ACROMIOCLAVICULAR JOINT AND CORACOCLAVICULAR LIGAMENTS

The acromioclavicular joint is small and intrinsically
unstable. It is thus easily subluxated. This is seen commonly
in rugger players who present with a painful 'bump' over the
joint. Pain settles in a few weeks with rest and function is
restored. A 'bump' however persists.

Complete acromioclavicular dislocation only occurs when
the coracoclavicular ligaments are torn. Now the clavicle
'flies' high and the shoulder droops. The deformity is ugly
and function impaired. A surgical repair is advisable.
Comparison radiographs will show the increased gap
between coracoid process and clavicle.

Technical considerations
Several operations have been described for repair of
complete acromioclavicular dislocation. The author favours
the transfer of coracobrachialis and short head of biceps to
the clavicle, a reliable procedure whether the injury is early
or late.

DISLOCATIONS OF THE STERNOCLAVICULAR JOINT

This is an uncommon injury. Usually the medial end of the clavicle dislocates forwards. Usually it can be pushed back and in some cases it can be held there by a pad stuck down by strapping. However in many cases it recurs and becomes permanent. Operations have been described for repair of chronic dislocation but the majority of cases do not require this.

Occasionally the dislocation occurs backwards where the clavicle may press on the trachea. This is a rarity but may require open reduction.

DISLOCATION OF THE SHOULDER

Practical anatomy
The majority of dislocations are anterior. Note that here there is a space for the dislocated humeral head to drift medially (subcoracoid) leaving the acromion process as the most lateral part of the shoulder. Much more rarely the dislocation is posterior. Here there is no space to move medially and the humeral head is still lateral but now posterior and palpable in the infraspinous fossa.

Pathology
In younger patients the capsule is strong and the dislocation usually occurs by stripping the labrum glenoidale and attached capsule off the bone leaving a permanent defect into which further dislocations can occur.

In older patients the capsule is burst apart. This will heal after reduction. Recurrent dislocation is thus less common but stiffness may be a problem.

Cause
The majority of injuries are due to indirect violence. Occasionally the shoulder may be dislocated by muscular contraction during convulsive episodes.

Who gets it?
Adults, young or old.

Clinical diagnosis
This is easy. An history and signs of injury plus visible and

palpable evidence of the absence of the humeral head from where it should be gives the diagnosis. The shoulder has a square instead of rounded shape (Fig 17).

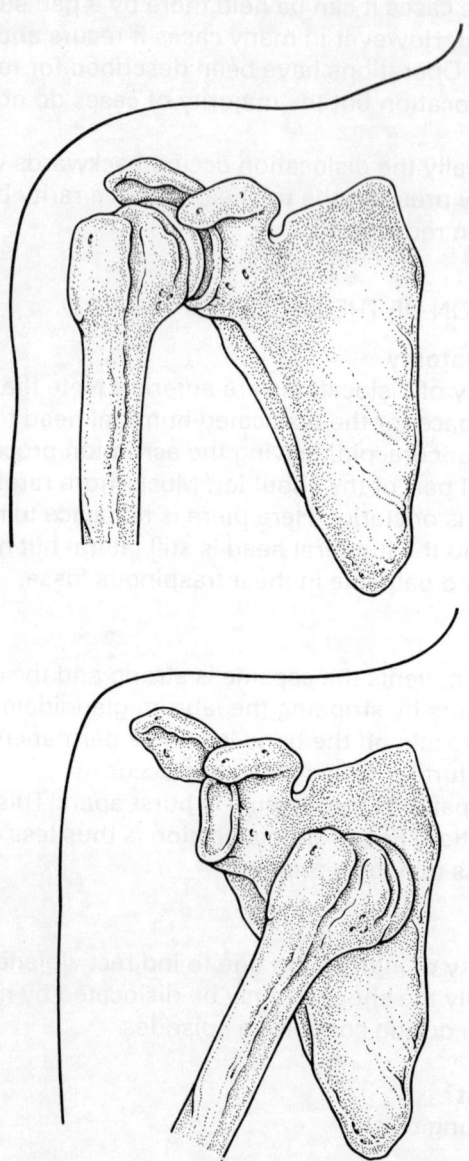

Fig. 17 Note how the shoulder becomes square after an anterior dislocation.

Radiographs in two planes confirm diagnosis.

Complications

A. *Early*
1. The axillary nerve may be damaged. Happily the vital structures in the axilla are not commonly damaged.
2. The shoulder capsule is badly damaged and there may be associated fractures.

B. *Late*
1. Stiffness. This may occur despite vigorous physiotherapy.
2. Recurrent dislocation. This indicates permanent damage to the capsule or capsular attachment to the glenoid and may require surgical repair.

Posterior dislocation

This injury is important for two reasons:

First it may be caused by muscle pull during a convulsive episode. Think of this if there is no definite story of injury.

Second it may be difficult to diagnose radiologically. The humeral head does not move medially and therefore on an anteroposterior radiograph it may not appear to be dislocated. Usually a lack of concentricity of the two articular surfaces is apparent. The humeral head has a symmetrical drumstick appearance and the superimposed greater tuberosity may appear as a 'cyst'.

However, clinical diagnosis is easy. The shoulder is not square but the humeral head is missing from its normal anterior position.

Treatment of anterior dislocation of the shoulder

The dislocation is reduced under general anaesthesia or under sedation with intravenous diazepam or similar drug.

With modern anaesthesia muscle relaxation is good and the ancient Hippocratic method of reduction is as good as any. The operator's stockinged foot is placed in the axilla and traction is applied to the semi-abducted arm.

The student may be required to be able to describe the manoeuvre attributed to Kocher. This was useful when speedy anaesthesia was not readily available, but is of less value nowadays. The stages of this time honoured manoeuvre are as follows:

1. The elbow is flexed to a right angle and traction in the line of the humerus is applied.
2. The humerus is rotated externally by use of the forearm.
3. The humerus is adducted across the trunk.
4. The humerus is internally rotated.
   Reduction by any method should be confirmed radiologically.

The limb is rested in a sling for up to two weeks after which active exercises are encouraged.

INJURY TO THE ROTATOR CUFF

This structure is very elastic, which allows the wide excursion of movement of the shoulder and is intimately related to several tendons which run through and help to stabilise the shoulder. Inflammation of or injury to these tendons gives rise to various clinical features.

Degeneration of the cuff occurs with increasing age and sudden strain upon the joint may cause rupture of the degenerate area — often containing the tendon of a specific muscle. The most important of these injuries is the supraspinatus tear.

Minor tears lead to 'supraspinatus tendonitis' and major tears render the patient incapable of initiating abduction of the shoulder. Plain radiographs may show calcification but are usually normal. Contrast medium arthrography may aid diagnosis.

Major tears in active fit people may require repair.

FRACTURES OF THE SURGICAL NECK OF THE HUMERUS (Fig. 18)

Cause
Usually direct violence due to fall onto the shoulder.

Who gets it?
Usually middle aged to elderly people, often female.

Diagnosis
History and signs of injury as expected. All fractures of the

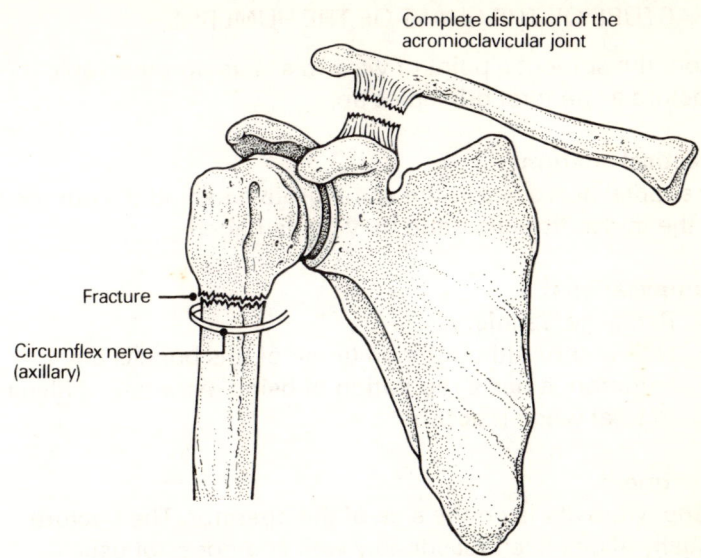

Fig. 18 1. Fracture of the surgical neck of the humerus.
        2. Complete acromio-clavicular dislocation.

upper humerus are accompanied by massive bruising of the upper arm. The seeming absence in some cases of severe pain may be due to impaction of the fracture.

Treatment
Immobilize for 3 weeks with body bandage and collar and cuff sling. Then commence physiotherapy.

In young patients there may be a need for manipulative reduction or even open reduction. Children may sustain a similar injury through the capital epiphysis, a fracture separation.

Complications
1. Rarely the axillary nerve may be damaged.
2. Stiffness is almost inevitable and some or all glenohumeral movement may be lost. Patients compensate well with scapulothoracic movement.

Communication with patient
Warn patient early that it may be difficult to mobilize the shoulder fully.

FRACTURE OF THE SHAFT OF THE HUMERUS

From the student's point of view this is an unremarkable fracture as general principles apply.

Practical anatomy
The radial nerve lies in the spiral groove behind the humerus in the midshaft region and may be damaged.

Complications
1. Radial nerve injury.
2. Non-union. Although non union of this bone is not common, it has a reputation of being extremely difficult to treat when it occurs.

Treatment
Happily gravity is on the side of the operator. The fracture usually aligns itself reasonably well and does not usually shorten. Occasionally manipulation under anaesthesia may be necessary.

Most cases can be treated by seating the patient, supporting the wrist with the elbow flexed and allowing the humerus to hang down by the patient's side. Wool is placed in the axilla and the arm is bandaged to the trunk. Plaster slabs can be stuck on to the bandaging as a shell and moulded to maintain alignment. Alternatively a U-slab may be used, also with the wrist supported in a collar and cuff sling. Some surgeons prefer a hanging cast. Occasionally open reduction and internal fixation may be required using a plate or intramedullary nail.

SUPRACONDYLAR FRACTURE OF THE HUMERUS (Fig. 19)

What makes this fracture so important clinically and so beloved of examiners? It is the importance and number of possible complications.

Supracondylar fractures occur in adults and may require conservative treatment, internal fixation or even skeletal traction. However, it is this fracture in childhood which holds the main interest.

Diagnosis
The child has a fall and presents with pain and a markedly

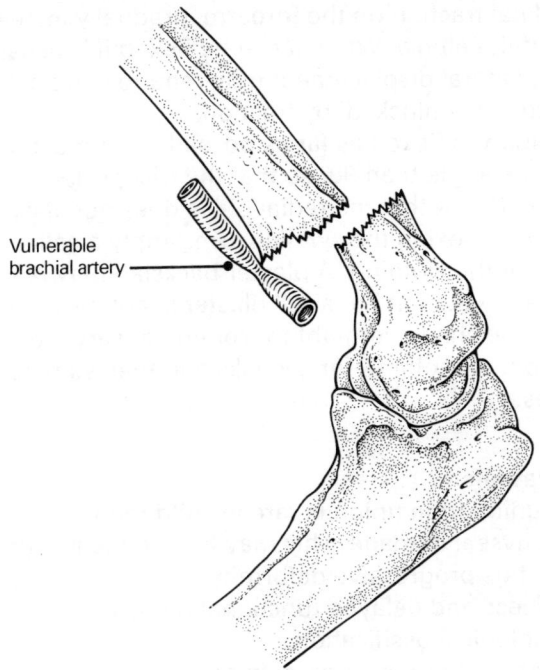

Vulnerable brachial artery

Fig. 19 Supracondylar fracture of the humerus.

swollen elbow. There is the usual reluctance to use the arm or to have it moved.

The fracture may be undisplaced, osteochondral and difficult to see or displaced posteriorly.

X-rays may at times be difficult to interpret, in which case comparison radiographs of the normal elbow aid diagnosis.

Practical anatomy
Note the position of the triceps muscle. When this taughtens in flexion it acts as a natural splint to a fracture displacing posteriorly.

Note the vulnerability of the brachial artery and median nerve.

Like the shoulder, the elbow has an elastic capsule which does not tolerate injury well.

Treatment
The fracture is manipulated under general anaesthesia with

longitudinal traction on the forearm, gradually increasing flexion of the elbow. When it can be flexed it is usually reduced. Lateral displacement may require correction when the fracture is 'unlocked' by traction.

The elbow is flexed as far as possible — it must be to a more acute angle than 90° so that the triceps 'locks' the reduction. Check that the radial pulse does not disappear through overflexing the swollen arm. Apply a collar and cuff sling under the clothing. A plaster backslab may reassure the parents and yourself but a full plaster is not necessary.

Admit the child overnight for routine observation of circulation. Immobilize for 3 weeks and then start active exercises.

Complications
1. Malunion (non union is rare in childhood).
2. Epiphyseal damage. This may lead to inequal growth and thus progressive deformity.
3. Stiffness and delayed functional recovery.
4. Pathological ossification.
5. Damage to nerves (Immediate)
                    (Late) — usually caused by
                              progressive deformity.
6. Damage to blood vessels.
7. Osteoarthrosis (late).
8. Reflex sympathetic dystrophy (rare in children).

Ischaemia of the forearm and hand following supracondylar fracture in childhood.
Despite the normally good collateral circulation in the upper limb, following this injury the forearm and hand can be ischaemic as a result of:

— Arterial injury with or without thrombosis.
— Arterial spasm.
— Gross intracompartmental swelling.
The clinical signs are:
— Absent pulses.
— Pallor.
— Poor capillary return.
— Excessive pain.
— Inability to permit full passive extension of the fingers.

By the time one sees loss of sensation or paralysis the diagnosis has been too long delayed. In grossly neglected cases gangrene may occur.

Treatment
Preventative: Anticipation and observation prevent this being overlooked.

Active: Remove all bandages, splints etc. Reduce the fracture immediately. Do not overflex a badly swollen arm.

If circulation is not restored in a few minutes summon surgical aid.

The surgeon will decompress the forearm surgically. If this fails to restore circulation a direct exploration of the brachial artery will be required.

Volkmann's ischaemic contracture
This is an entity much loved by examiners.

Following ischaemia of the forearm a block of tissue in the depths of the flexor compartment dies. The skin and superficial muscles survive. The necrotic deep flexors fibrose and contract creating a clawing of all digits.

FRACTURE OF THE LATERAL CONDYLE OF THE HUMERUS

This fracture is important for two reasons:

First it may be underestimated because much of the fragment in young children is cartilaginous. The fracture involves the capitellum, part of the epiphyseal plate and part of the lateral condylar mass. Second the fracture may lead to mal-union or non-union of the fragment. Either eventuality is associated with progressive deformity.

Treatment is along conventional lines.

FRACTURE OF THE OLECRANON

This is a direct impact injury usually treated by internally fixing the olecranon.

Technical considerations
Displaced olecranon fractures are best treated by open reduction and internal fixation with the intention of mobilizing the elbow early. Olecranon screws or tension band wiring may be used.

DISLOCATION OF THE ELBOW

This injury is caused by indirect violence.

It is a serious injury with severe damage to the elbow capsule.

The dislocation is almost always posterior and may be associated with minor fractures of adjacent bones.

The close proximity of major vessels and nerves necessitates careful examination and observation following this injury.

Treatment

Reduction should be performed early as follows:

The patient is placed supine with the arm flexed across the chest. Under general anaesthesia the elbow is flexed gently. Pressure is applied to the olecranon posteriorly until reduction occurs. The arm is rested in a plaster cast with the elbow at a right angle (Fig. 20) for three weeks, after which energetic active exercises must be encouraged. Physiotherapists must be discouraged from stretching the elbow passively.

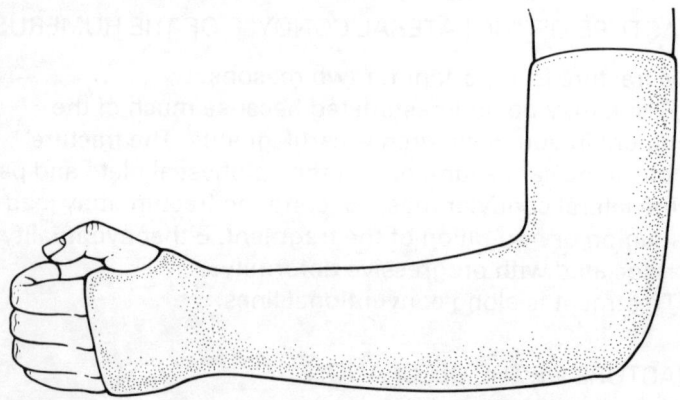

Fig. 20 Full length arm plaster neutral rotation and elbow at 90 degrees.

Complications
1. Vascular injury.
2. Joint stiffness.
3. Myositis ossificans.

FRACTURE OF THE RADIAL HEAD

This is an indirect violence injury. Signs are not impressive but tenderness over the radial head is constant.

Radiographs show the fracture.

Treatment is simple. Immobilize the elbow for two weeks and then commence physiotherapy. If the radial head is severely comminuted excision of the fragments may be the best treatment.

Communication with patient
Warn the patient that full extension will be difficult to achieve after this injury.

FRACTURES OF THE RADIUS AND ULNA

Practical anatomy
The radius and ulna not only connect the hand to the upper arm but they allow the specialized movements of pronation and supination in which the radius rolls around the ulna. Note that the radius is curved for this purpose and note that the two bones are intimately connected by the superior and inferior radio-ulnar joints. The radial head rolls on the capitellum.

Important significance of these facts
1. An injury to the forearm virtually always involves the two bones, or one bone plus one radio-ulnar joint. The only exception is a direct violence injury to the ulna such as might be sustained when lifting the arm to ward off a blow.

   The student must therefore think of injuries to the forearm as double injuries. Hence X-rays of forearm fractures should include the wrist and the elbow.
2. It is important to maintain the correct shape and length of the radius and ulna in order to preserve pronation and supination.

FRACTURES OF THE SHAFTS OF BOTH BONES

These are not remarkable injuries.

In children it is usual to try to treat them conservatively

unless displacement is severe. In adults because of the poor capacity for remodelling it is preferable to err on the side of internally fixing both bones.

Two fractures attract the attention of examiners by virtue of their eponyms, and the fact that they illustrate the double injury concept.

The Galeazzi fracture (Fig. 21)
Fracture in the distal half of the radial diaphysis plus subluxation of the inferior radio-ulnar joint. The fracture is difficult to treat conservatively and internal fixation of radius is usually required.

The Monteggia fracture (Fig. 21)
Here there is a fracture of the shaft of the ulna with dislocation of the radial head. Fixation of the ulna is essential for maintenance of reduction of the dislocated radial head.

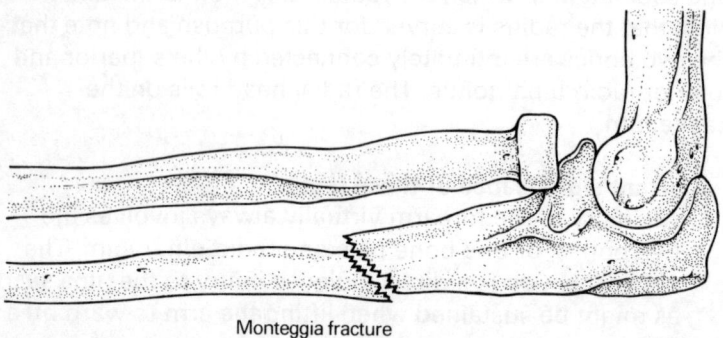

Monteggia fracture

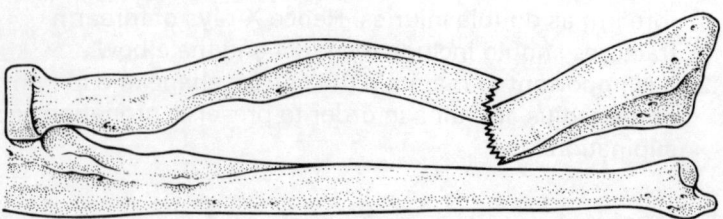

Galeazzi fracture

Fig. 21

Technical considerations

1. *Manipulation of fractures* of the forearm is conveniently done with the elbow flexed and the forearm suspended from the fingers by an assistant. Gravity will assist maintenance of the reduction.

Note that in fractures proximal to the insertion of pronator teres, the proximal fragment will tend to lie in some supination.

2. *Long arm plasters* for fractures of the forearm should be oval in section and thus flattened antero-posteriorly by the operator in the forearm section. 'Round' plasters allow the bones to fall inwards towards each other (Fig. 22).

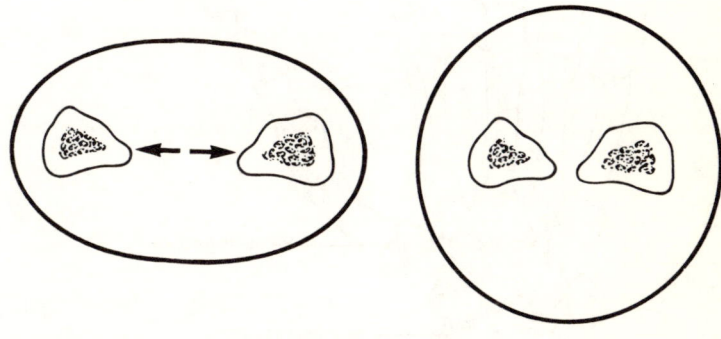

Fig. 22 An oval or flattened plaster cast keeps the radius and ulna apart.

3. A variety of *internal fixation devices* may be used. Intramedullary nailing has its place but most surgeons prefer plating. Whatever plate is used it is always certain that a six hole plate is better than a four hole plate. Semitubular plating has been popular but is often difficult to apply to bones of variable shape and also the plates tend to obscure the view of the bone on subsequent radiographs.

4. *In children* if internal fixation has reluctantly to be performed, little more than a bone suture is required. There is no need for sophisticated plating.

FRACTURES OF THE DISTAL END OF RADIUS

The Colles fracture (Fig. 23)

You must know this one as it is probably the commonest fracture of all.

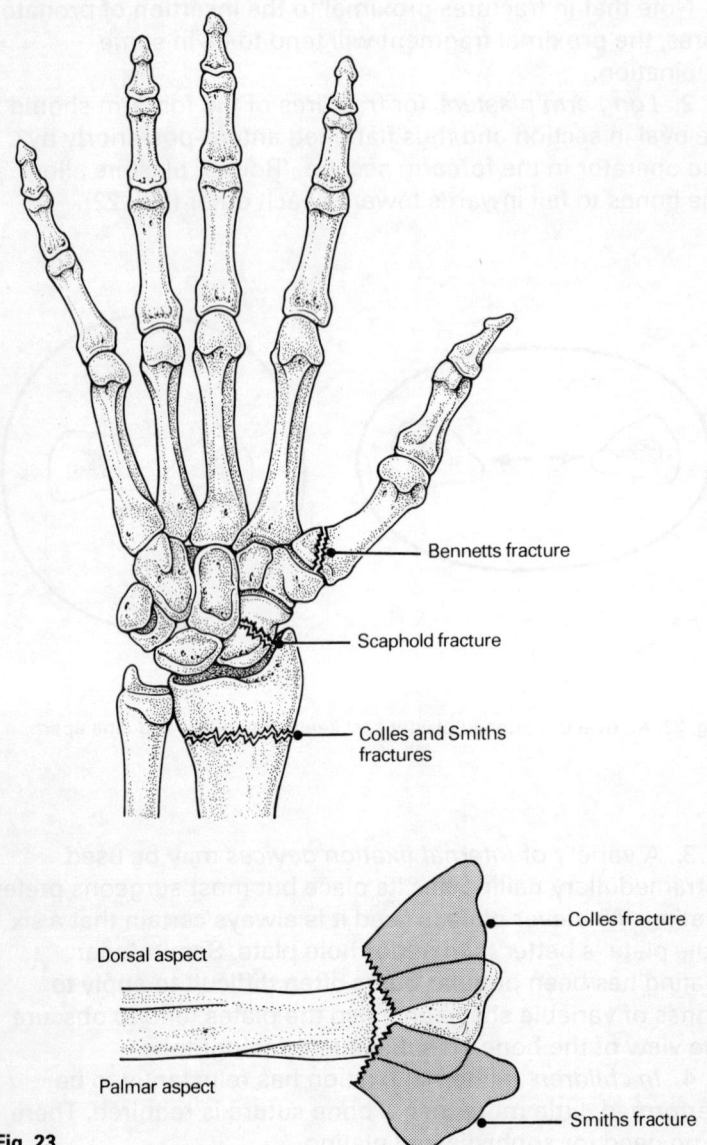

Bennetts fracture

Scaphold fracture

Colles and Smiths fractures

Colles fracture

Dorsal aspect

Palmar aspect

Smiths fracture

Fig. 23

It follows the rules. The radius fractures in its distal 3 cms with accompanying damage to radio-ulnar joint.

The classic displacement is threefold:

— The distal fragment tilts towards the dorsum.
— The distal fragment shifts towards the dorsum.
— The distal fragment shifs towards the radial side.

These displacements give the classic 'dinner fork' shape (Fig. 24A).

In point of fact the fractures are often comminuted and impacted.

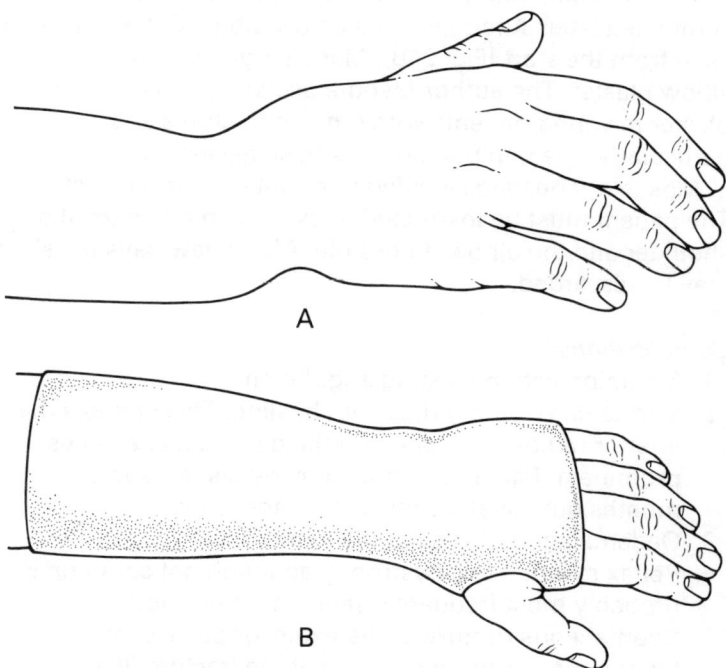

Fig. 24 (A) The typical 'Dinner fork' deformity of Colles fracture associated with radial and dorsal displacement.
(B) Colles plaster.

Who gets this fracture?
It is mainly a fracture of middle aged and elderly patients.

How do they get it?
They fall on the outstretched hand. If you think about it, this is a dorsiflexion-supination injury.

Treatment
Undisplaced or minimally displaced fractures of the distal
end of the radius merely require immobilization in a below
elbow plaster, after which care is the same as for a true
Colles fracture.

A Colles fracture with significant displacement requires
manipulation under general or local anaesthesia. The
fracture is disimpacted by traction and by exaggeration of
the dorsal tilt. The distal fragment is now levered over the
proximal, flexed and pronated. A plaster slab is applied
moulded to maintain this flexion and pronation. This may be
completed later. Alternatively a below elbow Colles plaster is
used from the start (Fig. 24B). Many surgeons use an above
elbow plaster. The author favours use of an above elbow
plaster in young patients with difficult fractures and
particularly if remanipulation has been necessary.

Most surgeons are satisfied to elevate the arm in a sling.
The patient must be instructed to exercise the fingers, the
shoulder and the elbow if possible. After a few days the sling
may be discarded.

Complications
1. Malunion with persisting angulation.
2. Shortening of the radius with healing. This disrupts the
   inferior radio-ulnar joint and the distal ulna becomes
   prominent. Pain in this area may persist for some
   months but usually settles spontaneously.
3. Oedema and stiffness of the hand.
4. Reflex sympathetic dystrophy although not common is
   probably most frequently seen after this injury.
5. Spontaneous rupture of the extensor pollicis longus
   tendon may occur after union of the fracture. It is
   probably even more common after undisplaced
   fractures.
6. Median nerve compression in the distorted carpal tunnel
   may produce the symptoms of carpal tunnel syndrome.
   Mild symptoms are quite frequent but it is unusual for
   surgical decompression to be required.

Communication with patient
Warn the patient that the wrist is unlikely to be exactly the
same shape as the other. Explain about radial shortening

which is not preventable and its effect on the radio-ulnar joint. At the same time encourage the patient by giving an excellent prognosis for function, provided they exercise hard.

The Smiths fracture (Fig. 23)
This is another beloved eponym and therefore important to students. The usage (slightly inaccurately) really covers two fractures. One is the reversed Colles fracture and the other is an anterior marginal fracture of the distal end of the radius with the distal fragment carrying the carpus anteriorly with it.

There is some discussion about the mechanism of this injury. Some cases are due to a fall onto the dorsum of the flexed wrist, such as might occur when a motor cyclist goes over his handlebar. However, the anterior marginal fracture appears to be a flexion-pronation injury.

Treatment
The general principles of treatment are similar to those of a Colles fracture but the reduced fracture is more stable in supination. Hence it is customary to use an above elbow plaster to hold the forearm supinated.

The fracture often occurs in young patients and the outcome is less favourable than in the case of Colles fractures. Because of this some surgeons prefer to treat difficult fractures by open reduction and plating.

FRACTURE SEPARATION OF THE DISTAL RADIAL EPIPHYSIS

This fracture occurs in children and corresponds to the Colles fracture in adults.

The epiphysis slips dorsally usually taking with it a small metaphyseal fragment.

Treatment is the same as for a Colles fracture but immobilization is not required for more than 4 weeks in the majority of cases.

GREENSTICK FRACTURES OF THE DISTAL RADIUS

This is probably the commonest site for 'greenstick'

fractures in childhood. The deformity is similar to a Colles fracture and the distal fragment needs to be held flexed and pronated. It is here that the use of a curved plaster may provide 'three point' correction of the deformity.

Beware the 'springy' greenstick fracture that redeforms within the plaster. In such cases it may often be better to use an above elbow plaster with pronation and 'three point' fixation of the forearm. After 2 weeks the long plaster can be changed to a short one. Union is sound by 4 weeks.

INJURIES TO THE CARPUS

Severe injuries to the carpus occur rarely with various combinations of dislocations and fractures. These require expert attention and often considerable disability results.

DISLOCATION OF THE LUNATE BONE (Fig. 25)

This injury may occur when a fall occurs onto a hand already extended. The lunate is squeezed out to lie anteriorly to its normal position.

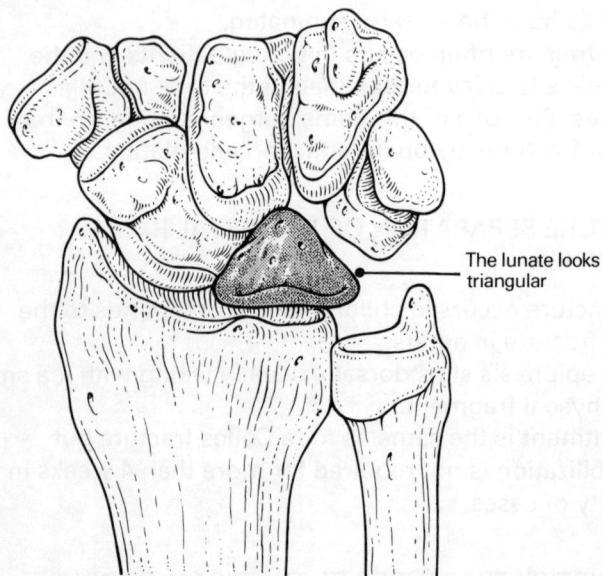

The lunate looks triangular

Fig. 25 Dislocation of the lunate bone.

The diagnosis is usually made radiologically. The lunate on an antero-posterior radiograph normally has a rectangular shape. When dislocated it is distinctly triangular (Fig. 25). Once this is spotted, careful inspection of a lateral film will show its abnormal rotated anterior position.

Treatment is by manipulation under anaesthesia followed by immobilization in a plaster cast. With traction on the hand, direct pressure is applied over the lunate in an attempt to push it back. If this fails open reduction may be required and late cases may be treated by excision of the lunate.

Complications
1. The notable complication is that of avascular necrosis of the lunate because of damage to its blood supply.
2. Osteoarthrosis of the wrist.
3. Median nerve compression.

FRACTURE OF THE SCAPHOID BONE (Fig. 26)

Practical anatomy
The scaphoid is one of those odd bones where the blood supply comes in from distal to proximal. Hence fractures across the body of the scaphoid may render the proximal fragment avascular.

Clinical features
1. The fracture occurs as a result of a fall on the outstretched hand.
2. A painful, swollen wrist with tenderness mainly in the anatomical snuffbox suggests the diagnosis.
3. The initial radiograph may fail to show the fracture. When this diagnosis is suspected, always ask for special 'scaphoid' views of the wrist. Even then the radiograph may be negative.

    Therefore the fracture must be treated on clinical grounds. A repeat X-ray at 2 weeks will probably show the fracture.
4. The fracture is treated in a plaster which includes the metacarpus and the thumb as far as the interphalangeal joint (Fig. 26). Apply the plaster as if the hand were holding a small glass of beer. The plaster is usually retained for six weeks in the first instance.

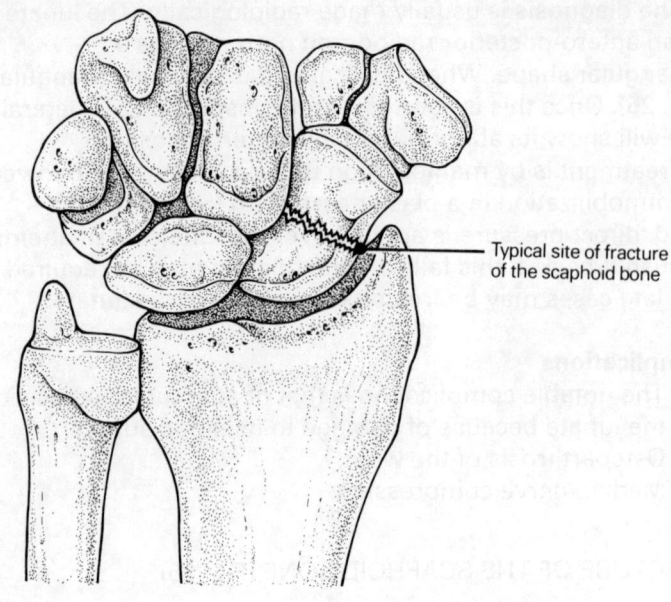

Typical site of fracture
of the scaphoid bone

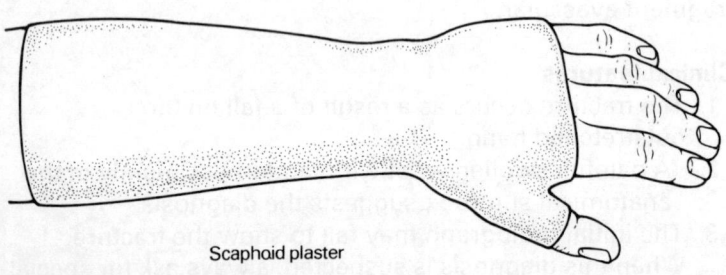

Scaphoid plaster

Fig. 26

Note that fractures of the tuberosity of the scaphoid are much less serious than fractures of the body and usually heal in less than 6 weeks.

Complications
1. Avascular necrosis of the proximal fragment.
2. Delayed union and non-union.

Union may be delayed but by 6 months it should be clear that non-union is present. This may be symptomless in which case it is not essential to interfere. If pain is present some form of bone grafting or fixation of the fracture should be attempted.
3. Osteoarthrosis of the wrist joint.

FRACTURE OF THE TRIQUETRUM

This injury is associated with pain and tenderness at the back of the wrist.

A 'flake' of bone is visible dorsally on the lateral radiograph.

Immobilization in a plaster cast for a few weeks is all that is required.

BENNETTS FRACTURE (see Fig. 23)

This is an eponym which survives and must therefore be learnt.

The fracture is oblique involving the ulnar side of the base of the 1st metacarpal bone. It enters the joint and in many cases is really a fracture-dislocation.

Treatment should be by manipulation and immobilization in a plaster cast similar to a scaphoid plaster. However, it is essential to extend the 1st metacarpal bone by moulding the plaster over felt pads. Note it is not the thumb but the 1st metacarpal that must be extended. If adequate reduction cannot be achieved by conservative means then percutaneous transfixation or open reduction and pinning or screwing of the fracture must be performed.

A transverse fracture of the base of the 1st metacarpal bone can also occur. This is not a Bennetts fracture. It is usually possible to treat this by manipulation and a scaphoid-type plaster.

GENERAL PRINCIPLES IN MANAGEMENT OF HAND INJURIES

The joints of the hand are vulnerable to oedema and stiffness and indeed oedema leads to stiffness. A united fracture is useless if the hand has lost its mobility. Hence:

1. Prevent oedema by elevation. Serious injuries require admission of the patient with formal elevation of the hand in a roller towel.
2. Encourage early movement. As a rule of thumb, the small joints of the hand should not remain unused for longer than 7–10 days.
3. Immobilize fractures for the minimum time essential.
4. Beware of crush injuries associated with fractures. Stiffness and oedema are a special problem in the crushed hand.
5. The collateral ligaments of the metacarpo-phalangeal joints are stretched in flexion and those of the interphalangeal joints are stretched in extension. Hence the ideal way to immobilize the damaged hand to prevent joint stiffness would be with the fingers straight but flexed at the metacarpo-phalangeal joints. Note that the popular 'boxing glove' bandaging often has the fingers in the reverse state which is not desirable. It is understood that it is not always possible to immobilize the hand in the ideal position but the dangers of a poor position must be avoided if possible.
6. Hand injuries must not be regarded as trivial injuries. Ideally follow up should be at a special clinic where expert advice is possible.
7. Injuries to the small joints of the hand often cause discomfort for many weeks. Mild swelling and pain persist. Reassurance of the patient and encouragement to continue use of the hand will ensure a satisfactory outcome.

FRACTURES OF THE METACARPAL BONES

These fractures may be caused by direct violence or by 'punching' injuries with the fist closed.

Undisplaced fractures may be treated with a light plaster slab and light strapping of the affected digit to its neighbour. Mobilization can be commenced immediately that pain allows.

Displaced fractures may need manipulation, or even internal fixation but this is not common.

Compound fractures of the hand require expert advice initially.

FRACTURE OF THE NECK OF THE FIFTH METACARPAL BONE

This is a frequent injury, usually caused by a misdirected punch. The distal fragment angulates towards the palm.

Minor displacement requires little treatment. Strapping the little finger to the ring finger and allowing movement is all that is required.

Severe displacement will call for manipulation under anaesthesia. The fracture is then held by splinting the little finger in flexion around a small roll of gauze. A malleable splint may also be used. Note that this fixation may well lead to stiffness and it should not be prolonged.

The fracture tends to heal with slight loss of prominence of the relevant knuckle and a bump on the dorsum of the hand. Function, however, is excellent even with slight persisting deformity.

FRACTURES OF THE PHALANGES

Practical anatomy
The proximal phalanx is surrounded by delicate and complex flexor tendons and extensor tendons. The lumbrical and interosseus muscles are inserted into the extensor hood on the dorsum. Damage to these or interference with their movement will cause loss of function.

Rotational deformities of the fingers may pass unnoticed when the finger is extended. However, when flexion occurs a rotational deformity will cause the finger to cross the palm and interfere with the flexion of its neighbour.

Treatment
On the whole, undisplaced fractures may be satisfactorily treated by strapping of the injured finger to its neighbour.

Displaced fractures may require manipulation and immobilization on a splint (padded aluminium splints are usually favoured). Compound fractures and displaced fractures of the proximal phalanx require special attention and often require internal fixation.

Fractures of the terminal tuft of the distal phalanx should be ignored and any soft tissue injury treated on its merit.

Fractures involving the interphalangeal joints themselves may need special attention and temporary internal fixation may be required.

DISLOCATIONS OF THE METACARPOPHALANGEAL AND INTERPHALANGEAL JOINTS OF THE HAND

These are nearly all due to hyperextension injuries. The distal bone dislocates posteriorly.

Reduction can usually be achieved by gentle traction and pressure over the head of the proximal bone anteriorly. After reduction has been confirmed by X-ray, strapping to the adjacent finger and immediate mobilization is all that is required.

Occasionally the proximal bone may 'button hole' the capsule and be irreducible. Open reduction is required.

MALLET FINGER INJURY

This injury is really an avulsion of the insertion of the extensor tendon into the base of the distal phalanx. It may involve a flake fracture or may be through the tendinous insertion. In general it is easier to manage the cases with an avulsed flake of bone.

The injury is caused by stubbing the finger when it is actively extended. Forced passive flexion causes the avulsion.

The finger adopts a position in which the distal phalanx is flexed. Some evidence of injury to the dorsum of the distal interphalangeal joint is often visible.

Treatment is by immobilization of the distal two phalanges of the finger in a 'mallet finger' splint. Immobilization may need to be continued for six weeks. However, even if healing does not occur, disability is minimal.

ULNAR COLLATERAL LIGAMENT RUPTURE OF THE FIRST METACARPOPHALANGEAL JOINT

This injury is mentioned because it is often overlooked and it is a disabling injury because pinch grip is impaired.

Thus if a patient presents with a painful swollen joint at

the base of the thumb after injury it is advisable to test the integrity of this ligament. Examine it in extension of the joint and compare it with the normal side.

Early complete rupture is best repaired as soon as possible. Chronic or neglected cases are often seriously inconvenienced with persisting pain and weakness. Various methods of repair are possible but in severe cases arthrodesis of the joint gives the surest result.

Ligament injuries

GENERAL PRINCIPLES FOR TREATING LIGAMENT INJURIES

1. *Partial tears* of a ligament may be expected to heal with 3–6 weeks adequate immobilization.

2. *Complete tears* may be associated with permanent instability of a joint. It is better therefore to make the diagnosis early. Often an injured joint (for example a tear of the medial ligament of the knee) may be so painful that the patient will not tolerate attempts to examine and to take strain radiographs of the joint. In such cases it is better to examine the joint under anaesthesia than to miss instability.

3. *A complete tear with demonstrable instability* requires early surgical repair. In practice we are thinking mainly of ankle and knee.

4. *Chronic injuries* (i.e. usually improperly diagnosed initially) may require sophisticated surgical repairs beyond the scope of this discussion.

5. Try to exclude *associated injuries* such as meniscus tears in the knee or extensive capsular damage.

LIGAMENT INJURIES TO THE KNEE JOINT

Soft tissue injuries to the knee are often multiple and early diagnosis is difficult. Combination injuries occur such as the classic medial ligament, medial meniscus and anterior cruciate ligament injury. The ligaments are intimately related to the joint capsule and capsular injuries are commonly associated. Certain clinical entities are usually described.

Tear of the medial ligament
Here an abduction strain on the tibia ruptures the medial ligament (often in association with other injuries as described).

The medial ligament is a long structure and may rupture at its upper end, at the joint line or below the joint line.

Clinically the patient presents with a painful swollen knee with tenderness maximal over the site of the tear. Pain may not allow demonstrable opening of the knee when a valgus strain is applied. However, if this injury is suspected it is worth performing an examination under anaesthesia. In partial tears a painful tense effusion may require aspiration.

Complete rupture should be repaired early followed by immobilization for six weeks in a plaster cylinder. Partial tears may be treated conservatively for three weeks in a similar plaster. It is advisable to follow immobilization with a period of physiotherapy and to remember the possibility that other structures may have been damaged giving rise to further symptoms.

Tear of the lateral ligament
It is doubtful whether isolated injuries of this ligament occur. Management of instability on the lateral side of the knee is similar to that on the medial. Instability is rare because the biceps femoris tendon which is inserted into the head of the fibula helps to stabilize the lateral side of the knee.

Tear of the cruciate ligament
The anterior cruciate ligament is usually torn by hyperextension or forward movement of the tibia on the femur in the flexed knee. The posterior cruciate ligament is torn by a force drawing the tibia backwards on the femur when the knee is in flexion.

These lesions are often associated with a feeling of giving way and instability in the knee. Examination with the patient supine, the knee flexed and the muscles relaxed will show that the tibia can be pulled forward or displaced backwards on the femur more than can be shown on the normal side. The clinical presentation is often influenced by associated injuries.

An 'isolated' cruciate ligament tear does not usually require specific treatment. Repairs are not reliably successful. It is preferable to concentrate on building up the patients' quadriceps muscles by physiotherapy. Most patients learn to live happily with this damaged knee.

The concept of rotatory instability
It used to be said that giving way and locking of the knee

were either due to loose bodies in the knee or tears of the menisci. More recently it has been shown that the combination of ligament tears plus capsular tearing may allow rotatory instability. This implies that the tibia subluxates forward on the femur momentarily when the tibia is rotated on the femur. The patient experiences a sensation of giving way whenever he twists on the knee in a particular direction.

Examination of the knee may show evidence of old injury or cruciate laxity but it requires considerable experience to be able to perform the clinical tests for rotatory instability.

The student is asked to remember that the condition exists and by thinking of it to avoid indescriminate removal of menisci. The patient with rotatory instability will certainly not be improved by meniscectomy.

LIGAMENT INJURIES TO THE ANKLE JOINT

Sprained ankle

As has been previously described, the anterior fibres of the lateral ligament of the ankle may be torn during an inversion injury to the ankle.

Usually pain, swelling and tenderness are well localized below and in front of the lateral malleolus.

The condition may be treated in a variety of ways. Simple bandaging and strapping help most cases. Sportsmen are often treated energetically with physical medicine techniques. More severe cases may benefit from the use of eversion strapping or even a short spell in a walking plaster.

Chronic sprain of the ankle

This clinical entity refers to a condition where, following an ankle injury, the patient experiences repeated episodes of going over on the ankle (i.e. instability) associated with pain and swelling often lasting a few days.

Some of these cases can be shown to have frank lateral ligament insufficiency but the majority do not have such dramatic pathology.

Investigation includes plain radiographs of the ankle and the use of stress inversion films. The latter technique involves the taking of antero-posterior radiographs of both ankles when they are held in forced inversion. The abnormal side can be compared with the normal and if there is gross 'opening' of the ankle on the lateral side, then it is reasonable to assume that the lateral ligament is incompetent.

The average case can usually be treated with a course of physiotherapy including inversion-eversion exercises.

Complete rupture of the lateral ligament
This is an uncommon injury and is often not diagnosed until it is in the chronic stage.

An inversion sprain followed by very severe pain, bruising and swelling may give a clue to the diagnosis. Plain radiographs are usually normal but sometimes an avulsion flake fracture may be seen. Stress films (which may require an anaesthetic) will show 'opening' of the ankle with a talar tilt.

Most cases can be satisfactorily treated in a below knee walking plaster for six weeks. Some surgeons are enthusiastic about early surgical repair. Chronic cases demonstrating instability will require a surgical reconstruction of the lateral ligament.

Meniscus tears

GENERAL PRINCIPLES OF DIAGNOSIS AND TREATMENT
OF MENISCUS TEARS IN THE KNEE JOINT

1. The patient gives a story of injury usually with an
   element of 'twisting of the knee'.
2. The pain may or may not be well localized but if it is the
   diagnosis is made easier.
3. The patient is initially disabled, i.e. he does not continue
   playing football.
4. The knee is swollen and painful often with tenderness
   over the torn cartilage.
5. The knee will settle down gradually if rested or
   immobilized and the patient may think all is well.
6. The second or chronic phase of the symptom pattern
   now appears. The classic presentation is of recurrent
   episodes of pain and swelling with giving way or locking
   of the knee.
7. Medial meniscus tears are 5–6 times as common as
   lateral meniscus tears and are easier to diagnose as they
   more often give a 'classic' story.
8. The plain radiograph is likely to be normal.
9. Doubtful cases may be investigated radiographically by
   contrast medium arthrography or the knee may be
   directly inspected through an arthroscope.
10. A severely torn meniscus does not heal and therefore
    meniscectomy is usually necessary. It is probable that
    minor injuries to the menisci often remain undiagnosed.

Pathology of meniscus tears (Fig. 27)
Tears of the semilunar cartilage are usually inflicted by
twisting forces when the knee is partially flexed bearing
weight and often with a valgus or varus strain in addition.
     There is a line roughly centrally down the long axis of a
meniscus where tearing predominates. Complete tearing

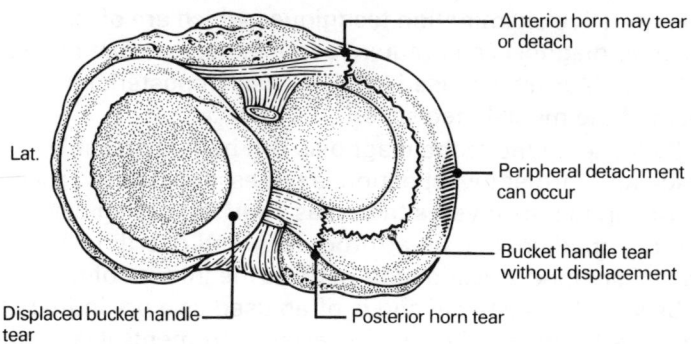

Anterior horn may tear or detach

Lat.

Peripheral detachment can occur

Bucket handle tear without displacement

Displaced bucket handle tear

Posterior horn tear

Fig. 27 Injuries to the menisci.

virtually divides the meniscus into two. The inner section can then flip over (like the action of a bucket handle), obstruct the joint and give rise to the features of a 'bucket handle' tear. Less severe injuries cause tags either anteriorly or posteriorly and frequently horizontal cleavage lesions may be found.

Clinical features
The patient gives a story of injury. Often the injury is well described but sometimes it is vague. Examination in the acute phase reveals merely a painful swollen knee with tenderness over the joint line on the damaged side. Sometimes the knee is locked which makes the diagnosis almost certain. Care must be taken to distinguish this injury from a ligament tear which may require urgent surgery. The radiographs are negative.

Usually the knee is treated with some form of pressure bandaging and gradually settles down. When the patient becomes more active again the classical symptoms of episodes of pain, swelling, giving way and locking appear.

Examination in the chronic phase will show definite physical signs. The quadriceps muscles are usually wasted, there is likely to be an effusion in the knee, there is tenderness over the affected meniscus in the joint line. The examiner may be fortunate enough to witness the knee locked but a much more frequent finding is the loss of the last few degrees of extension and hyperextension. This is often described as a 'springy block' to extension, which is a good description of the physical finding. There are various manipulative examination techniques which are of lesser value to diagnosis and require some expertise. One of these is the McMurray test used for diagnosis of posterior horn tears of the medial meniscus.

By these methods the diagnosis can be fairly reliably made and further investigation is not essential in all cases. However, in recent years there has been increasing use of contrast medium and air arthrography and of arthroscopy. The last named investigation permits the interior of the joint to be visualized directly and is often used as a preliminary to formal arthrotomy. By use of special instruments it is possible to perform surgical procedures in the knee joint under arthroscopic vision without having to open the joint formally.

Treatment of the acutely locked knee consists of manipulating it under general anaesthesia. This should not be regarded as anything more than a temporary measure which allows reasonable comfort until the patient can be investigated and treated as above.

Index